D0904967

Arthritis

Fight It
with
the Blood
Type Diet®

Also by Dr. Peter J. D'Adamo with Catherine Whitney

Eat Right 4 Your Type: The Individualized Diet Solution to Staying Healthy, Living Longer, and Achieving Your Ideal Weight

Cook Right 4 Your Type: The Practical Kitchen Companion to Eat Right 4 Your Type

Live Right 4 Your Type: The Individualized Prescription for Maximizing Health, Metabolism, and Vitality in Every Stage of Your Life

Eat Right 4 Your Baby: The Individualized Guide to Fertility and Maximum Health During Pregnancy, Nursing, and Your Baby's First Year

Eat Right 4 Your Type Complete Blood Type Encyclopedia

Blood Type O: Food, Beverage and Supplement Lists

Blood Type A: Food, Beverage and Supplement Lists

Blood Type B: Food, Beverage and Supplement Lists

Blood Type AB: Food, Beverage and Supplement Lists

Dr. Peter J. D'Adamo's Eat Right 4 Your Type Health Library

Diabetes: Fight It with the Blood Type Diet®

Cancer: Fight It with the Blood Type Diet®

Cardiovascular Disease: Fight It with the Blood Type Diet®

DR. PETER J. D'ADAMO

WITH CATHERINE WHITNEY

Dr. Peter J. D'Adamo's

Eat Right for Your Type

4

Health Library

Arthritis

Fight It with the Blood Type Diet®

G. P. PUTNAM'S SONS

NEW YORK

ıllP

G. P. Putnam's Sons
Publishers Since 1838
a member of
Penguin Group (USA) Inc.
375 Hudson Street
New York, NY 10014

Library of Congress Cataloging-in-Publication Data

D'Adamo, Peter, date.
Arthritis : fight it with the blood type diet /
Peter J. D'Adamo with Catherine Whitney.
p.   cm.
(Eat right 4 (for) your type health library)
Includes index.
ISBN 0-399-15227-X
1. Arthritis—Diet therapy.   2. Blood groups.
I. Whitney, Catherine.   II. Title.
RC933.D335   2004   2004044393
616.7'220654—dc22

Printed in the United States of America
1   3   5   7   9   10   8   6   4   2

This book is printed on acid-free paper. ∞

DEDICATED TO MY PATIENTS,
WHOSE COURAGE IN THE FACE
OF CHRONIC PAIN IS
A DAILY INSPIRATION

Acknowledgments

THIS BOOK OFFERS THE BEST THAT NATUROPATHIC MEDICINE AND blood type science have to offer in the prevention and treatment of arthritis. It has been a collaborative process, and I want to express my deep thanks to the people who have been involved in its creation.

I am most grateful to Martha Mosko D'Adamo, not only my partner in life and in parenting but also my partner in bringing the valuable wisdom about blood type to the world. Martha daily provides love, support, insight, and inspiration to all of my endeavors.

Catherine Whitney, my writer, and her partner, Paul Krafin, are invaluable word masters who have once again captured exactly the right tone in tackling this complex topic.

My literary agent and friend, Janis Vallely, always takes time to listen and advise. Her quiet guidance and personal support make the work possible.

I would also like to acknowledge others who have made significant contributions to this book: my colleague Bronner Handwerger, N.D., whose research and clinical abilities helped make this book comprehensive and practical; Heidi Merritt, who continues to make an important contribution to the work; John Harris, whose knowledge and input have been invaluable; Laura Mittman, N.D., FIFHI, who has been such a big help in my efforts to educate other professionals; and Catherine's agent, Jane Dystel, who provides support.

Amy Hertz, my editor at Riverhead/Putnam, has been the force behind the success of all the blood type books, and she continues to guide my work with dedication and skill.

As always, I am extremely grateful to the wonderful staffs at Riverhead Books and Putnam. They have been tireless and enthusiastic, and their efforts have made it possible to continue bringing this important work to the market.

PETER J. D'ADAMO, N.D.

Contents

New Tools to Fight Arthritis

THE BLOOD TYPE DIET CAN BENEFIT EVERYONE. YOU don't have to be sick to see the effects. But most of the people who come to my clinic or contact my Web site are dealing with a serious chronic disease or have received a distressing medical diagnosis. They want to know how they can hone the general guidelines of the Blood Type Diet to target their illness. Dr. Peter J. D'Adamo's Eat Right 4 (for) Your Type Health Library has been introduced with these people in mind.

Arthritis: Fight It with the Blood Type Diet allows you to take full advantage of the medicinal benefits of eating and living according to your blood type. If you think of the standard Blood Type Diet as the foundation, the guidelines in this book provide a more targeted overlay for people who want to act aggressively to treat arthritis. These dietary and lifestyle adaptations, individualized by blood type, supply additional ammunition to your arthritis-fighting arsenal. They attack the problem at its source, restoring balance to your immune system and eliminating the factors that trigger inflammation and cause the destruction of joints. These strategies give you the tools you need to restore health, reduce pain, and increase mobility.

Here's what you'll find that's new:

- A disease-fighting category of blood type–specific food values, the **Super Beneficials,** emphasizing foods that have medicinal properties for arthritic conditions.
- A more detailed breakdown of the **Neutral** category to limit foods that are known to have less nutritional value or can exacerbate your condition. Foods designated **Neutral: Allowed Infrequently** should be minimized or avoided.
- Detailed supplement protocols for each blood type that are calibrated to support you at every stage. They include an **Anti-Inflammatory Protocol** and three adjunct protocols for **Arthritis Pain Relief, Joint Repair,** and **Surgery Recovery.**
- A **4-Week Plan** for getting started that emphasizes what you can do right now to improve your condition and start feeling better right away.
- Plus: many strategies for success, quizzes, checklists, and the answers to the questions most frequently asked about arthritis at my clinic.

The chemistry of blood type continues to provide important clues to the biological and genetic mechanisms that control health and disease. In more than twenty-five years of research and clinical practice, I have successfully treated thousands of patients with arthritis, autoimmune inflammatory diseases, and related conditions. Increasingly, medical doctors and naturopaths throughout the world are applying the blood type principles in their practices, with remarkable results.

I urge you to talk to your physician about the benefits of incorporating individualized, blood type–specific diet, exercise, and lifestyle strategies into your current plan. I am confident that using the guidelines in this book will start you on the road to recovery. Take the step now, and use your blood type to your best advantage.

Why Blood
Type Matters

YOU ARE A BIOLOGICAL INDIVIDUAL.

Have you ever wondered why some people are constitutionally frail and susceptible to infection while others seem naturally hardy? Why are some people able to lose weight on a particular diet while others fail? Why do some people age rapidly and show early signs of deterioration while others are full of vitality into their later years?

We are all different. A single drop of your blood contains a biochemical signature as unique to you as your fingerprint. Many of the biochemical differences that make you an individual can be explained by your blood type.

Your blood type influences every facet of your physiology on a cellular level. It has everything to do with how you digest food, your ability to respond to stress, your mental state, the efficiency of your metabolic processes, and the strength of your immune system.

You can greatly improve your health, vitality, and emotional balance by knowing your blood type and by incorporating blood type–specific diet and lifestyle strategies into your health plan.

Be the biological individual you were meant to be!

What's Your Blood Type– Arthritis Risk?

Blood Type O Quiz
Are You Arthritis-Prone?

General Factors

The following factors are known to contribute to an individual's risk for developing arthritis. Answer yes or no to each question.

		yes	no
1.	Are you over the age of 60?	☐	☐
2.	Is there a history of arthritis in your family?	☐	☐
3.	(Women) Does/did your mother have osteoarthritis?	☐	☐
4.	Are you obese (more than 30% overweight)?	☐	☐
5.	Have you suffered repeated joint injuries in adulthood?	☐	☐
6.	Are you a "weekend athlete"?	☐	☐
7.	Do you have an autoimmune disease?	☐	☐
8.	Do you regularly engage in work or other activities that place stress upon weight-bearing joints?	☐	☐
9.	Have genetic tests revealed markers for particular autoimmune diseases (e.g., ankylosing spondylitis)?	☐	☐
10.	Do you have periodontal disease or other chronic dental problems?	☐	☐

Blood Type O–Specific Factors:

The following factors are known to specifically influence Blood Type O's risk for arthritis and related conditions. Answer yes or no to each question.

1. Do you consume a high-carbohydrate, low-protein diet?   ☐ yes   ☐ no
2. Do you regularly consume wheat or corn products?   ☐ yes   ☐ no
3. Are you a coffee drinker?   ☐ yes   ☐ no
4. Do you regularly consume dairy foods?   ☐ yes   ☐ no
5. Do you lead a sedentary lifestyle that includes little aerobic exercise?   ☐ yes   ☐ no
6. Do you suffer from depression?   ☐ yes   ☐ no
7. Do you have gastrointestinal problems, such as ulcers?   ☐ yes   ☐ no
8. Do you have eat a lot of nightshade foods (tomatoes, potatoes, etc.)?   ☐ yes   ☐ no
9. Do you have allergies or hay fever?   ☐ yes   ☐ no
10. Are you a non-secretor? (see page 36)   ☐ yes   ☐ no

Scoring: Add the number of "yes" responses in each list. Give yourself two points for each "yes" answer in General Factors and one point for each "yes" answer in Blood Type O–Specific Factors. Your score is based on the total:

18–30: High Risk You are very likely to develop an arthritic condition, or you already have one. Take immediate action with adherence to the Blood Type Diet and modify the factors that are in your control.

8–17: Moderate Risk If you make some diet and lifestyle changes and begin an appropriate exercise program, you may avoid arthritis or related conditions in the future. Refer to your blood type section to determine which actions you must take.

0–7: Low Risk Your risk for developing arthritis or a related condition is low. Keep it that way by adhering to the Blood Type Diet and lifestyle plan.

Blood Type A Quiz
Are You Arthritis-Prone?

General Factors

The following factors are known to contribute to an individual's risk for developing arthritis. Answer yes or no to each question.

1. Are you over the age of 60? ☐ yes ☐ no
2. Is there a history of arthritis in your family? ☐ yes ☐ no
3. (Women) Does/did your mother have osteoarthritis? ☐ yes ☐ no
4. Are you obese (more than 30% overweight)? ☐ yes ☐ no
5. Have you suffered repeated joint injuries in adulthood? ☐ yes ☐ no
6. Are you a "weekend athlete"? ☐ yes ☐ no
7. Do you have an autoimmune disease? ☐ yes ☐ no
8. Do you regularly engage in work or other activities that place stress upon weight-bearing joints? ☐ yes ☐ no
9. Have genetic tests revealed markers for particular autoimmune diseases (e.g., ankylosing spondylitis)? ☐ yes ☐ no
10. Do you have periodontal disease or other chronic dental problems? ☐ yes ☐ no

Blood Type A–Specific Factors

The following factors are known to specifically influence Blood Type A's risk for arthritis and related conditions. Answer yes or no to each question.

1. Do you consume a high-protein, high-fat diet? ☐ yes ☐ no
2. Do you eat wheat once or twice a day? ☐ yes ☐ no
3. Do you eat dairy foods every day? ☐ yes ☐ no
4. Do you have a high-stress lifestyle? ☐ yes ☐ no
5. Do you often have trouble sleeping and wake feeling tired? ☐ yes ☐ no

6. Do you easily succumb to infections, colds, and flu? ☐ yes ☐ no
7. Do you lead a sedentary lifestyle? ☐ yes ☐ no
8. Do you eat red meat on a regular basis? ☐ yes ☐ no
9. Is there a history of heart disease in your family? It can be a related risk factor for Blood Type A. ☐ yes ☐ no
10. Are you a non-secretor? ☐ yes ☐ no

Scoring: Add the number of "yes" responses in each list. Give yourself 2 points for each "yes" answer in General Factors and 1 point for each "yes" answer in Blood Type A–Specific Factors. Your score is based on the total:

18–30: High Risk You are very likely to develop an arthritic condition, or you already have one. Take immediate action with adherence to the Blood Type Diet and modify the factors that are in your control.

8–17: Moderate Risk If you make some diet and lifestyle changes and begin an appropriate exercise program, you may avoid arthritis or related conditions in the future. Refer to your blood type section to determine which actions you must take.

0–7: Low Risk Your risk for developing arthritis or a related condition is low. Keep it that way by adhering to the Blood Type Diet and lifestyle plan.

Blood Type B Quiz
Are You Arthritis-Prone?
———

General Factors

The following factors are known to contribute to an individual's risk for developing arthritis. Answer yes or no to each question.

1. Are you over the age of 60? ☐ yes ☐ no
2. Is there a history of arthritis in your family? ☐ yes ☐ no
3. (Women) Does/did your mother have osteoarthritis? ☐ yes ☐ no

4. Are you obese (more than 30% overweight)? ☐ yes ☐ no
5. Have you suffered repeated joint injuries in adulthood? ☐ yes ☐ no
6. Are you a "weekend athlete"? ☐ yes ☐ no
7. Do you have an autoimmune disease? ☐ yes ☐ no
8. Do you regularly engage in work or other activities that place stress upon weight-bearing joints? ☐ yes ☐ no
9. Have genetic tests revealed markers for particular autoimmune diseases (e.g., ankylosing spondylitis)? ☐ yes ☐ no
10. Do you have periodontal disease or other chronic dental problems? ☐ yes ☐ no

Blood Type B–Specific Factors

The following factors are known to specifically influence Blood Type B's risk for arthritis and related conditions. Answer yes or no to each question.

1. Do you consume a high-carbohydrate, low-fat diet? ☐ yes ☐ no
2. Do you avoid dairy foods, especially cultured varieties like yogurt? ☐ yes ☐ no
3. Do you regularly consume wheat or corn products? ☐ yes ☐ no
4. Do you regularly consume any of the following foods: chicken, buckwheat, peanuts, lentils? ☐ yes ☐ no
5. Do you lead a sedentary lifestyle that includes little aerobic exercise? ☐ yes ☐ no
6. Are your work and/or personal life exceptionally stressful? ☐ yes ☐ no
7. Do you have a history of viral infections? ☐ yes ☐ no
8. Do you have a history of urinary or reproductive tract infections? ☐ yes ☐ no

9. Do you have an autoimmune disease? ☐ yes ☐ no
10. Are you a non-secretor? ☐ yes ☐ no

Scoring: Add the number of "yes" responses in each list. Give yourself 2 points for each "yes" answer in General Factors and 1 point for each "yes" answer in Blood Type B–Specific Factors. Your score is based on the total:

18–30: High Risk You are very likely to develop an arthritic condition or you already have one. Take immediate action with adherence to the Blood Type Diet and modify the factors that are in your control.

8–17: Moderate Risk If you make some diet and lifestyle changes and begin an appropriate exercise program, you may avoid arthritis or related conditions in the future. Refer to your blood type section to determine which actions you must take.

0–7: Low Risk Your risk for developing arthritis or a related condition is low. Keep it that way by adhering to the Blood Type Diet and lifestyle plan.

Blood Type AB Quiz
Are You Arthritis-Prone?

General Factors
The following factors are known to contribute to an individual's risk for developing arthritis. Answer yes or no to each question.

1. Are you over the age of 60? ☐ yes ☐ no
2. Is there a history of arthritis in your family? ☐ yes ☐ no
3. (Women) Does/did your mother have osteoarthritis? ☐ yes ☐ no
4. Are you obese (more than 30% overweight)? ☐ yes ☐ no
5. Have you suffered repeated joint injuries in adulthood? ☐ yes ☐ no
6. Are you a "weekend athlete"? ☐ yes ☐ no

7. Do you have an autoimmune disease?   ☐ yes ☐ no
8. Do you regularly engage in work or other
    activities that place stress upon weight-
    bearing joints?   ☐ yes ☐ no
9. Have genetic tests revealed markers for
    particular autoimmune diseases
    (e.g., ankylosing spondylitis)?   ☐ yes ☐ no
10. Do you have periodontal disease or other
    chronic dental problems?   ☐ yes ☐ no

Blood Type AB–Specific Factors

The following factors are known to specifically influence Blood Type AB's risk for arthritis and related conditions. Answer yes or no to each question.

1. Do you consume a high-protein, high-fat diet,
    with little or no soy protein or cultured dairy?   ☐ yes ☐ no
2. Do you eat wheat once or twice a day?   ☐ yes ☐ no
3. Do you regularly consume any of the following
    foods: chicken, buckwheat, lentils?   ☐ yes ☐ no
4. Do you eat red meat more than twice a week?   ☐ yes ☐ no
5. Do you lead a sedentary lifestyle, with little
    aerobic, strengthening, or flexibility exercise?   ☐ yes ☐ no
6. Do you suffer from depression?   ☐ yes ☐ no
7. Do you consume fewer that 4–5 servings of
    vegetables each day?   ☐ yes ☐ no
8. Do you easily succumb to infections, colds,
    and flu?   ☐ yes ☐ no
9. Is there a history of joint disease in your family? ☐ yes ☐ no
10. Are you a non-secretor?   ☐ yes ☐ no

Scoring: Add the number of "yes" responses in each list. Give yourself 2 points for each "yes" answer in General Factors and 1 point for each "yes" answer in Blood Type AB–Specific Factors. Your score is based on the total:

18–30: High Risk You are very likely to develop an arthritic condition, or you already have one. Take immediate action with adherence to the Blood Type Diet and modify the factors that are in your control.

8–17: Moderate Risk If you make some diet and lifestyle changes and begin an appropriate exercise program, you may avoid arthritis or related conditions in the future. Refer to your blood type section to determine which actions you must take.

0–7: Low Risk Your risk for developing arthritis or a related condition is low. Keep it that way by adhering to the Blood Type Diet and lifestyle plan.

PART I

Blood Type and Arthritis: A Basic Primer

The
Dynamics
of Arthritis

SEVERAL YEARS AGO, WHILE I WAS SPENDING A LOT OF TIME at my computer, both of my shoulders froze up. The condition seemed to come out of the blue. One morning I woke up to find that any movement of my upper body caused painful spasms that radiated across my upper back and neck. If I turned the wrong way, a sharp pain cut across the front of my shoulders, so severe that I had to hold them tightly. Not only was I unable to work at my computer, treat patients, or drive a car, I was also unable to perform even the most mundane tasks without excruciating pain.

At first I thought I was suffering from muscle strain, but after several days had passed with no improvement, I realized it was more serious. In fact, my condition had a name—"frozen shoulder syndrome," technically known as adhesive capsulitis. The conventional treatments for severe frozen shoulder syndrome include corticosteroid injections and even surgery. However, since I had often used the Blood Type

Diet with great success in treating patients for joint conditions, it seemed logical that I begin with my own best "medicine."

As you might imagine, I am pretty serious in my adherence to the diet for my type, which is Blood Type A. But since I'm relatively healthy, I have never been as rigid in my own compliance as I suggest that people suffering from chronic illnesses be. So, two weeks into my painful journey with double frozen shoulders, I took a careful look at my diet. I eliminated many NEUTRAL foods, including wheat, and concentrated almost exclusively on foods that were BENEFICIAL for Blood Type A. The extra compliance paid off. Within seventy-two hours, my shoulders were "unfrozen," and my life returned to normal.

Having experienced it myself, I feel a new empathy for my patients who suffer debilitating joint pain. And I'm more convinced than ever that the Blood Type Diet can make a profound difference for so many of them.

The Complexity of Movement

THE HUMAN BODY has 120 joints—points in the body where bones connect to allow movement. Cartilage serves as cushioning at the ends of bones to allow for easy movement. It's a remarkable system, operating seamlessly thousands of times a day, whenever you pick up a pencil, get dressed, stand up from a sitting position, turn your head, raise a fork to your mouth, open a jar, reach into your pocket, or walk across a room. If you've never suffered from joint pain, these ordinary movements occur without thought. Arthritis changes everything. The simplest tasks become immensely difficult, and sometimes impossible. Arthritis makes young people feel old, and it robs the elderly of many of the last vestiges of their independence.

Arthritis can be a difficult disease to define. Although the word literally means joint (*arth*) inflammation (*itis*), it is a disease syndrome that includes more than one hundred conditions, with a variety of underlying causes. Arthritic conditions range from the deterioration of osteoarthritis to the systemic invasion of rheumatoid arthritis to the inflammatory effects of diseases like fibromyalgia and scleroderma. More than 45 million Americans suffer from arthritis.

The two most common forms of arthritis are osteoarthritis and rheumatoid arthritis. Osteoarthritis is the deterioration of cartilage in one or several joints. More than half of all osteoarthritis sufferers are over age sixty-five. Rheumatoid arthritis is a systemic inflammatory condition, attacking the synovium (the membranes surrounding joints). It is triggered by a dysfunction in the immune system and can occur at any age.

Osteoarthritis: Cartilage Deterioration

OSTEOARTHRITIS IS A DEGENERATIVE joint disease, mostly affecting cartilage, the slippery tissue that covers the ends of bones in a joint. Healthy cartilage allows bones to glide over one another and absorbs energy from the shock of physical movement. In osteoarthritis, the surface layer of cartilage breaks down and wears away. This allows bones under the cartilage to rub together, causing pain, swelling, and loss of motion of the joint. Over time, the joint may lose its normal shape.

Although osteoarthritis is associated with aging, it is not merely the inevitable result of "wear and tear." Many of my patients assume that all older people eventually get osteoarthritis, but that's far from the case. Rather, the course of osteoarthritis has several paths.

Much of the focus of current osteoarthritis research is on defining the genetic connection. Researchers suspect that genes play a role in 25 to 30 percent of osteoarthritis cases. A gene defect affecting collagen, an important component of cartilage, appears to be a key trigger in patients with an inherited kind of osteoarthritis that begins at an early age. The mutation weakens collagen protein, which may break or tear more easily under stress.

Researchers recently found that daughters of women who suffer from osteoarthritis of the knee have a significant increase in cartilage

breakdown, thus making them more susceptible to disease. This finding may be important in identifying people who are at risk for
osteoarthritis.

From the standpoint of prevention, it is clear that dietary and
lifestyle factors play a part in both the development of osteoarthritis
and its relief. Obesity and muscle weakness are often seen in osteoarthritis sufferers. Losing weight and embarking upon an appropriate exercise program can bring significant relief.

Studies also show that those who have repeated joint injuries in
young adulthood are more likely to develop osteoarthritis later in life.
These studies underscore the need for increased education about joint
injury prevention and use of proper sports equipment.

Rheumatoid Arthritis: Systemic Inflammatory Disease

RHEUMATOID ARTHRITIS IS an autoimmune disease that occurs
when the body's immune system attacks and damages the joints and
sometimes other organs. It usually follows a symmetrical pattern,
meaning that if one knee or hand is involved, the other one is, too.
Symptoms include swelling and stiffness in the joints, pain, fever, and
a purplish hue in the affected area. Rheumatoid arthritis is unlikely to
be due to a single cause, but rather to a combination of genetic and en-
vironmental factors that trigger an abnormal immune response. Possible
contributing factors include prior infection, food sensitivities, heavy
metal toxicity, a high-fat diet, hypothyroidism, and free radical damage.

The autoimmune event is triggered when white blood cells travel
to the synovium (a fluid-filled membrane that acts much like a shock absorber) and cause inflammation. The ensuing warmth, redness, swelling,
and pain in the joints are typical symptoms of rheumatoid arthritis.
Eventually, the disease destroys the cartilage that coats the end of the
bones. This narrows the joint space and eventually damages bone. The
surrounding muscles, ligaments, and tendons that support and stabilize
the joint also become weak and are unable to work normally.

In a properly functioning immune system, molecules, known as antibodies, are produced which are capable of recognizing the chemical structure of invading pathogens, such as viruses and bacteria. Antibodies are highly specific for antigens, which are unique markers on the surfaces of potential invaders. They trigger white blood cells to launch an attack against the invaders, aided by chemicals called the complement system.

Some of the most powerful antibodies in your body are those related to your ABO blood type—the reason transfusions of incompatible blood can be fatal. Many substances, such as bacteria, viruses, parasites, and some foods, actually resemble foreign blood type antigens, and it is the job of your blood type antibodies to recognize these intruders and target them for removal.

In rheumatoid arthritis and many related autoimmune diseases, a hyperactive inflammatory response plays a significant role in this process. Sensitization of the immune system, which can occur by inoculation with reactive food proteins, by infection, or even by one's own tissues, primes specialized antibody-producing cells called lymphocytes to manufacture antibodies, which target and tag offenders so that other cells of the immune system can scavenge and destroy them.

Individuals with rheumatoid arthritis have been shown to produce structurally different antibodies from individuals without rheumatoid arthritis.

Antibody molecules are usually comprised of two sections: a variable section that is altered to fit the particular antigen the antibody is being designed for, and a constant section that doesn't change and is the place that white blood cells can attach to and complete the killing. An antibody is very much like a plumber's wrench: There is the portion that can be adjusted to fit the particular nut that needs tightening or loosening, and the stable handle that the plumber grips.

In healthy individuals, the constant portion of the antibody molecule is normally comprised of long chains of a sugar called galactose. In rheumatoid arthritis, the galactose is replaced with another amino sugar called N-acetyl glucososamine (NAG). NAG is a preferred binder for many food proteins—in particular, lectins commonly found in wheat.

The Inflammatory Response

INFLAMMATION IS A POWERFUL systemic response, and as such is a force to be reckoned with. More people die of inflammatory diseases than all other disease processes combined; just ponder for a moment the huge number of medical conditions ending in "itis." Increasingly, scientists are learning that inflammation is a factor in many diseases not previously considered inflammatory. These include heart disease, diabetes, and Alzheimer's disease.

Although inflammation can do a lot of damage, its initial purpose is protective. Without an adequate inflammatory response by the body's cells, we would not survive for long, since the inflammatory response is necessary to fight infection and heal damaged tissue. The types of damage that induce inflammation include allergic reactions, tissue damage, bone fracture, and injuries due to cuts, burns, and infections. Virtually all of the white blood cells, as well as the blood-clotting platelets, are involved in the inflammatory response. The cells involved either contain or can produce more than one hundred chemical mediators of the inflammatory response.

Inflammation directs the elements of the immune system into damaged tissues by increasing the blood supply to the infected area and increasing the permeability of the tiniest blood vessels, the capillaries. This process allows larger molecules to migrate into an infected area. Most of the cells traveling to the site are scavenger cells, with Pac Man–like attributes. These cells engulf and digest offending microorganisms.

To trigger the inflammatory response, proteins called selectins mediate the binding of white blood cells to the walls of the blood vessels. This generates signals that initiate the inflammatory response. In the absence of selectins, inflammatory cells cannot adhere to activated cells lining the blood vessels when blood flow is sufficiently high. Thus, selectins initiate inflammation on the walls of blood vessels. Underproduction of selectins is equivalent to an immune deficiency, while overproduction can mimic many inflammatory diseases. Also involved in the inflammatory response are messenger proteins called cytokines, which induce the release of acute phase proteins, such as complement, and act as fever producers. Selectin levels are somewhat under the influence of diet, and their levels have been shown to induce histamine formation.

The chemical histamine plays a prominent role in some types of inflammation, including allergy. The antihistamine drugs that many people depend upon during an allergy season are acting effectively as anti-inflammatories by reducing the production of histamine.

The protracted process of inflammation can often be more harmful than the event that originally stimulated it. A system of such complexity, with so many different players, can be difficult to control. Many chemicals involved in the immune response are very caustic, as their main purpose is to kill the invader. However, if the reaction is intense, there can be a spillover of chemicals, resulting in damage to the tissues in the area.

In the process of waging an attack on foreign invaders, there is a buildup of immune complexes, an insoluble lattice network of antibodies bound to antigens in the bloodstream. Immune complexes are harmful when they accumulate and initiate inflammation. One of the major jobs of the complement system is "garbage removal." Complement helps remove immune complexes by making them soluble. They can then bind to red blood cells, which pass them on to scavenger cells for their ultimate removal. Low complement levels are characteristic of many inflammatory diseases, including rheumatoid arthritis.

Other Arthritic Diseases

THERE ARE MANY DISEASES that have arthritic effects. Most of them involve inflammatory autoimmune responses, although the picture is more complex than that. It is likely that most of these conditions stem from multiple factors.

Ankylosing Spondylitis

Ankylosing spondylitis is a chronic inflammatory type of arthritis that mainly affects the spine. Once thought to be part of rheumatoid arthritis, we now know that ankylosing spondylitis is related to rheumatoid arthritis but is a separate disease that affects men three to four times more than women.

The most common symptom of ankylosing spondylitis is lower back pain. Similar to rheumatoid arthritis, the pain is dull and aching at first. Many people will also experience pain in the legs, shoulders, buttocks, and the back of their knees. The ankle may be very tender in the spot where the tendon attaches to the bone. Often, a person with ankylosing spondylitis will also have an inflammation of the eye called iritis.

Ankylosing spondylitis is inheritable. A genetic marker called HLA-B27 establishes a predisposition to the disease. Ankylosing spondylitis is usually active for about ten years and may then level off. It can leave permanent damage to the spine, hips, or knees. People who develop ankylosing spondylitis as teenagers are more likely to have other types of arthritis and need hip replacement than those who develop it after age thirty.

There appears to be an association between individuals who cannot secrete their blood type and an increased risk of ankylosing spondylitis. For more information on the secretor system, see page 36.

Fibromyalgia

Fibromyalgia syndrome has had a long, if rather obscure, history as an illness. It is a complex, chronic condition that causes widespread pain and fatigue. The name fibromyalgia comes from "fibro" (fibrous tissues, such as tendons and ligaments), "my" (muscles), and "algia" (pain). Unlike arthritis, fibromyalgia does not cause pain or swelling in the joints themselves; rather, it produces pain in the soft tissues located around joints, skin, and organs throughout the body. Because the symptoms of fibromyalgia are so hard to pinpoint, it has been dubbed the "irritable everything" syndrome.

The pain of fibromyalgia usually consists of diffuse aching or burning described as "head to toe" and is often accompanied by muscle spasms. Its severity varies from day to day and can change location, becoming more severe in parts of the body that are used the most (e.g., the neck, shoulders, and feet). For some people, the pain can be intense enough to interfere with work and daily tasks, while others experience only minimal discomfort. Likewise, the fatigue of fibromyalgia varies from person to person, ranging from a mild, tired feeling to the exhaustion of a flu-like illness.

Fibromyalgia is not an easy disease to diagnose. The standard method involves digital palpitation of eighteen tender points. Approximately nine pounds of pressure is applied to a tender point, and if the patient indicates that the point is tender, it is considered positive. An official diagnosis of fibromyalgia requires eleven tender points.

Although the cause of fibromyalgia is not currently known, it is clear that there is a breakdown in the pain perception system in fibromyalgia patients, causing them to be extraordinarily sensitive to pain.

Recently, a great deal of interest has been directed at the neuroendocrine system and the abnormal status of such neurochemicals as calcitonin-gene-related peptide, noradrenaline, endorphins, dopamine, histamine, and gamma-aminobutyric acid (GABA). Hormones of the hypothalamus, pituitary, and adrenal glands are thought to be dysfunctional, too.

Sometimes the disease will first appear after an injury or illness such as a back injury, the flu, or Lyme disease. However, there is no specific evidence that an illness or an injury causes fibromyalgia.

There may be a link between depression and fibromyalgia. Depression may lead to changes in the chemistry of the brain and release substances that cause more sensitivity to pain, resulting in fibromyalgia.

Some studies have shown that both stress and poor physical condition may be factors in the cause of fibromyalgia. It is suspected that during times of stress the symptoms will be worse, and that the pain will subside during less stressful times.

There has been some data in the medical literature suggesting that an avoidance of wheat products may improve the conditions of some fibromyalgia sufferers. Some blood types are known to have immunologic problems from excessive wheat consumption.

Gout

Gout is a form of arthritis that occurs when crystals of uric acid accumulate in a joint, leading to the sudden development of pain and inflammation. Individuals with gout either overproduce uric acid or are less efficient at eliminating it. The big toe is the most commonly afflicted joint to accumulate uric acid crystals, although other joints may be affected.

Incidents of gout often develop very quickly, including swelling in the joints that lasts for about a week without treatment. The skin may be red and shiny around the affected joints. Uric acid crystals may cause lumps to form under the skin around the elbows, heels, or ears. The uric acid crystals that cause these lumps can also cause kidney stones.

There are many reasons why an episode of gout will appear, including drinking too much alcohol or eating certain kinds of food rich in purines, such as seafood, beans, sweetbreads, canned or processed gravies, and anchovies. Gout can also be triggered by stress, high blood pressure, and medical treatments, such as chemotherapy.

Infectious Arthritis

In some cases, arthritis can develop as part of a bacterial or viral infection. If a bacterial infection is involved, early diagnosis and treatment with antibiotics may relieve the arthritis symptoms and cure the disease. One form of infectious arthritis, called reactive arthritis, can develop following an infection of the lower urinary tract, intestines, or other organs. It is commonly associated with eye problems, skin rashes, and mouth sores. Parvovirus arthritis and gonococcal arthritis are examples of infectious arthritis. Symptoms of arthritis may also occur in Lyme disease, which is caused by a bacterial infection following the bite of infected deer ticks.

Evidence suggests that Blood Type B individuals may be somewhat protected genetically against developing reative arthritis, while non-secretors may have a higher risk.

Juvenile Chronic Arthritis

Nearly 300,000 children in America have some form of juvenile chronic arthritis (formerly called juvenile rheumatoid arthritis).

Juvenile arthritis is a chronic condition that causes inflammation in one or more joints and begins before the age of sixteen. It is the most common form of arthritis in children. Symptoms include pain, stiffness, swelling, and loss of function in the joints. The arthritis may be associated with rashes or fevers, and it may affect other parts of the body. Unlike adult rheumatoid arthritis, most children do not have a long-term disease, and they usually lead healthy lives as adults.

Psoriatic Arthritis

Psoriatic arthritis is an inflammatory arthritis associated with psoriasis, a chronic skin and nail condition. It often affects the joints at the ends of the fingers and causes changes in the fingernails and toenails.

Scleroderma

Also known as systemic sclerosis, scleroderma means "hard skin." It is a chronic autoimmune arthritic disease that primarily affects females who are thirty to fifty years old at onset. It is a serious illness that can target any part of the body and is often referred to as a "disease that turns people into stone," for the distinctive skin hardening that often occurs. The hardening typically affects the hands, causing the fingers to curl inward. In scleroderma patients, there is an excessive production of collagen (a fiberlike protein) in the involved areas of the skin or internal organs. The symptoms vary among individuals. Although there is no cure, early diagnosis and treatment can minimize the symptoms and prevent severe damage to organs and tissues.

Studies indicate that individuals with scleroderma have elevated antibodies to opposing blood types. For example, Blood Type A scleroderma sufferers have elevated levels of anti-B antibodies. These antibodies are believed to arise from the diet—specifically from plant foods that contain blood type antigens.

Sjögren's Syndrome

A chronic, systemic, inflammatory disorder of unknown cause, Sjögren's syndrome is often associated with rheumatic disorders sharing certain autoimmune features.

Sjögren's syndrome attacks mucous membranes. It can cause extremely dry eyes (sometimes described as the feeling of sand in the eyes or a burning sensation), dry mouth and throat, dental cavities from lack of saliva, enlarged glands, vaginal dryness, and fatigue, as well as joint pain, stiffness, and swelling. Less common symptoms include rashes, numbness, and inflammation of the lungs, kidneys, or liver.

A major risk factor for developing Sjögren's is being a postmenopausal woman. Other risk factors include having an autoimmune disease such as lupus, vasculitis, thyroid disease, or scleroderma, and/or a family member with Sjögren's. An association has been found between HLA-DR3 antigens, detected in the blood, and Sjögren's syndrome in Caucasians.

Systemic Lupus Erythematosus (SLE)

Systemic lupus erythematosus (SLE) is an inflammatory autoimmune disease that can involve joints, kidneys, and tissues. Symptoms of lupus include fever, skin rash, anemia, and joint disease. It is nine times more common in women, and more common still in African Americans, Hispanics, and Asians. It classically strikes after puberty and before menopause. Lupus is also related to abnormalities in the metabolism of estrogen, progesterone, and androgens, as well as a deficiency of immune modulators such as complement.

There are some genetic markers—HLA-B8, HLA-DR2, HLA-DR3—that may reveal significant risk for the development of lupus. These markers can be detected through DNA tests, using blood or body tissue.

Lupus is more common in Blood Type B individuals, and in other blood types is characterized by inappropiate levels of antibodies made in response to stimulation with the B antigen.

Tendonitis and Bursitis

Tendonitis is an inflammation of the tendons—tough cords of tissue that connect muscle to bone. It can be caused by overuse, injury, or arthritis-producing conditions. Symptoms include pain, tenderness, and a restriction in the movement of nearby joints. A related condition, bursitis, involves inflammation of the bursae—small, fluid-filled sacs that help reduce friction between bones and other moving structures in the joints. The inflammation may result from arthritis in the joint or injury or infection of the bursae. Bursitis produces pain and tenderness and may limit the movement of nearby joints.

Other Risks Associated with Arthritis

We know that arthritis can exert a systemic effect, and a major new study bears this out. Researchers at Brigham and Women's Hospital found that women with rheumatoid arthritis had twice the risk of heart attack compared to those without it. Those who had the joint condition for at least ten years faced triple the heart attack risks of nonsufferers. The study, based on nearly 28,000 women, is by far the largest to look at inflammation's role, and it shows that those with high levels are twice as likely as those with high cholesterol to die from heart attacks and strokes.

Doctors believe inflammation has many possible sources. Often, the fatty buildups that line the blood vessels become inflamed as white blood cells invade in a misguided defense attempt. Fat cells are also known to turn on these inflammatory proteins. Other possible triggers include high blood pressure, smoking, and lingering low-level infections such as chronic gum disease. Inflammation is thought to weaken the fatty buildups, or plaques, making them more likely to burst. A piece of plaque can then lead to a clot that can choke off the blood flow and cause a heart attack.

How Is Arthritis Diagnosed?

ALTHOUGH MOST FORMS of arthritis have symptoms in common, the ability to distinguish the precise condition and its underlying causes is the key to treatment.

Your physician will conduct a complete physical examination, including a urinalysis and complete blood count. X-rays, computed tomography (CT scan), or magnetic resonance imaging (MRI) may help detect cartilage damage. Additional tests may include:

Antinuclear antibody (ANA) This test checks blood levels of antibodies that are often present in people who have connective tissue diseases or other autoimmune disorders such as lupus. Since the antibodies react with material in the cell's nucleus (control center), they are referred to as antinuclear antibodies.

C-reactive protein test This is a nonspecific test used to detect generalized inflammation. Levels of C-reactive protein are often increased in patients with active disease such as rheumatoid arthritis.

Complement This test measures the level of complement, a group of proteins in the blood that involve proper immune function. A low blood level of complement is common in people who have active lupus.

Erythrocyte sedimentation rate (sed rate) As old as Hippocrates, this blood test is used to detect inflammation in the body. Higher sed rates indicate the presence of inflammation and are typical of many forms of arthritis, such as rheumatoid arthritis, ankylosing spondylitis, and many of the connective tissue diseases.

Hematocrit (PCV, packed cell volume) This test and the test for hemoglobin (a substance in the red blood cells that carries oxygen throughout the body) measure the number of red blood cells present in a sample of blood. A decrease in the number of red blood cells (anemia) is common in people who have inflammatory arthritis or another rheumatic disease.

Rheumatoid factor This test detects the presence of rheumatoid factor, an antibody found in the blood of most (but not all) people who have rheumatoid arthritis.

Synovial fluid examination Synovial fluid (fluid in the membranes surrounding joints) may be examined for white blood cells (found in people with rheumatoid arthritis and infections), bacteria or viruses (found in patients with infectious arthritis), or crystals in the joint (found in patients with gout or other types of crystal-induced arthritis). To obtain a specimen, the doctor injects a local anesthetic, then inserts a needle into the joint to withdraw the synovial fluid into a syringe. The procedure is called arthrocentesis, or joint aspiration.

Before you see a doctor, write down your symptoms and their duration and try to be as specific as possible. Typical symptoms might include swelling in one or more joints that has persisted for two or more weeks, a feeling of warmth and redness in a joint, constant or recurring pain or tenderness in a joint, stiffness around one or more joints upon rising that lasts an hour or more, deep fatigue, and flu-like symptoms accompanying joint swelling or aching.

Gather as much relevant information as you can. Have close relatives suffered from arthritis or autoimmune disorders? Have you had prior joint pain from injuries or infection? Have you recently had an injury or infection? Have you engaged in unusual physical activity or overexercised? Arrive at your physician's office armed with the information that will lead to the right diagnosis.

The Blood Type–Arthritis Connection

WHAT DOES YOUR BLOOD TYPE HAVE TO DO WITH YOUR risk for arthritis? Quite a bit, as it turns out. Your blood type is a key modulator of your digestive system, metabolic activity, and immunity. Think of it as your physiological balancing factor.

Blood Type and Immunity

EACH BLOOD TYPE is determined by the presence or absence of chemical markers called antigens, and each blood type antigen has a unique chemical structure. It is easy to remember your blood type antigen, as your blood type is named for it. Blood Type A has an A antigen on its red blood cells; Blood Type B has a B antigen; Blood Type AB has both an A and a B antigen; and Blood Type O has no (or "zero") antigen.

We can visualize the chemical structure of blood types an antennae of sorts, projecting outwards from the surface of our cells into deep space. These antennae are made from long chains of a repeating sugar called fucose, which by itself forms the O antigen of Blood Type O. Fucose also serves as the base for the other blood types, A and B. Blood Type A is actually the O antigen (fucose) plus a sugar named N-acetyl galactosamine added to its end. Blood Type B is fucose, plus a different sugar, named D-galactosamine, at the end. Blood Type AB is fucose plus N-acetyl galactosamine.

When a foreign antigen enters the body it provokes the activity of antibodies—specialized chemicals manufactured by the cells of the immune system. Antibodies attach and "tag" it in a manner that results in its disposal. The cells of our immune system manufacture countless varieties of antibodies, and each is specifically designed to identify and attach to one particular foreign antigen.

Most people carry antibodies against the antigens of the other blood types. These blood type antibodies are not there to complicate transfusions, but rather to protect your body against foreign substances, such as bacteria, viruses, parasites, and some plant foods that can actually resemble foreign blood type antigens. When your immune system encounters one of the substances resembling a blood type opposed to yours, it creates antibodies against it. This antibody reaction is characterized by a process called agglutination. That is, the antibody you create will attach to the antigen of the foreign substance, often linking two or more antigens together to create clumps of bacteria, viruses, etc.

Many foods contain proteins called lectins, which can bind to sugars (including blood type antigens) and thus agglutinate the cells of certain blood types but not others. That is why a food may be harmful to the cells of one blood type but beneficial to the cells of another. This discovery of the link between blood type and diet has significant implications for the prevention and management of arthritis.

Lectins and Arthritis: A Critical Reaction

YOUR BLOOD TYPE'S reaction to dietary lectins can trigger or amplify some forms of arthritis. While some lectins react with tissues of all blood types, many lectins are blood type–specific, in that they show a clear preference for one kind of sugar (the structural basis of blood type antigens) over another and mechanically fit the antigen of one blood type or another. This blood type specificity results in their attaching to the antigen of a preferred blood type, while leaving other blood type antigens completely undisturbed. At the cellular level, a common effect of lectins is to provoke the sugars on the surface of one cell to cross-link with those of another, effectively causing the cells to stick together and agglutinate, perhaps their most well-known effect. Not all lectins cause agglutination; many bacteria have lectinlike receptors that they use to attach to the cells of their host. Other lectins, called mitogens, cause a proliferation of certain cells of the immune system. But, in the most basic sense, lectins make things stick to other things.

Lectins activate autoantibodies in inflammatory and autoimmune diseases. For example, some studies show that the antibody produced in rheumatoid arthritis may require activation by wheat germ lectin. My own research has demonstrated that many cases of rheumatoid arthritis and fibromyalgia may stem from sensitivity to wheat—especially for Blood Type O individuals.

According to the *British Journal of Nutrition*, which published a recent review of the subject, strong evidence exists that dietary lectins play a significant role in autoimmune and inflammatory diseases. The authors of the study show that interaction between dietary lectins and the cells lining the intestines may unnecessarily "rev up" the immune system.

The key to the so-called "arthritis cure," which has gained popularity in recent years, may actually be that it chemically mimics the effects of a low-lectin diet. The two sugars used in the treatment, glucosamine and chondroitin, may have lectin-blocking actions. Some forms of glucosamine bind wheat germ lectin very effectively, while chondroitin replicates the Blood Type A antigen in very long linkages (polymerized). In either case, it is very likely that both function as sacrificial molecules, reacting with lectins to prevent them from reacting with the inflamed tissue. So, while Blood Type A may benefit from chondroitin, Blood Type O may find it counterproductive.

Your Blood Type Susceptibility

ALL BLOOD TYPES can suffer from arthritic conditions. However, individuals differ in the ways they get there, and one factor involves blood type. Much like separate roads might follow different routes to the same city, individual blood types contract arthritis by different means.

Blood Type O

Even though Blood Type O has a lower incidence of arthritis than Blood Type A, Blood Type O is more inflammation-prone than the other blood types. Thus, when Blood Type O does develop arthritis, it tends to be more aggressive. A key factor in Blood Type O's vulnerability to a range of inflammatory problems is the fucose sugar that acts as its blood type antigen. Fucose sugars serve as adhesion molecules for selectins, allowing the easy migration of white blood cells from the bloodstream into the areas of inflammation.

Blood Type O individuals who consume a lot of grains in their diet are adding to their autoimmune disease susceptibility. The lectins exacerbate the tendency for hyperimmunity, which is characteristic of autoimmune diseases.

The link between Blood Type O and rheumatoid arthritis may also be related to inflammation of the gut. It is a widespread clinical observation that inflammation of the gut is frequently associated with inflammation of the joints, and vice versa. In one study, evidence was provided that the interaction of dietary lectins with immune mediators triggered inflammation. Many times, an intolerance to a food lectin will develop after a bout of intestinal flu or some other form of gastroenteritis. This has been speculated to be the result of the intestinal inflammation "stripping away" the lining of the intestinal tract, uncovering the base tissue. The reaction of dietary lectins with intestinal cells (enterocytes) and immune cells (lymphocytes) may facilitate the movement of both dietary and gut-derived pathogens to peripheral tissues such as the joints. These, in turn, stimulate the immune system in those peripheral areas. In genetically susceptible individuals, this antigenic stimulation may ultimately result in molecular mimicry, a process where foreign peptides, similar in structure to those made by the body, cause antibodies to cross-react and attack the body's own tissues.

In one study of patients with rheumatoid arthritis, more than half were found to have peptic ulcers and/or erosions. Although a greater number of patients with ulcers and/or erosions were taking regular aspirin or indomethacin, a comparable number of patients with abnormal and normal endoscopies were using nonsteroidal anti-inflammatory drugs, such as ibuprofen. Seventy-six percent of these patients were Blood Type O. The conclusion is that not only is Blood Type O more likely to have stomach bacteria, but is also more likely to have inflammation from it. When taking anti-inflammatory medications that harm the stomach, Blood Type O is more likely to suffer from gastrointestinal complications.

Blood Types A and AB

Blood Types A and AB may be more susceptible to the deteriorating effects of arthritis. Repeatedly, studies show a preponderance of Blood Type A and a significant lack of Blood Type O among patients with osteoarthritis and other deteriorating conditions, such as spinal osteochondrosis.

Arthritis in Blood Types A and AB individuals tends to be mediated by the activity of adhesion molecules on the artery wall called selectins. Blood Types A and AB are known to have higher selectin levels than the other blood types. Selectins, and E-selectin in particular, are part of an amazing cellular process we are only now beginning to understand by which white blood cells migrate through the vascular lining into the tissues, often in response to injury or infection. Thus one of the prime "highways" to inflammation has a greater number of "exit ramps" in Blood Type A or AB individuals.

Several components of the diet are known to influence selectin levels. High animal protein diets further increase E-selectin, while a soy protein diet significantly lowers selectin levels. One important component of soy, the isoflavone genestein, inhibits enzymes necessary to increase selectins and other vascular adhesion molecules.

Blood Type B

The arthritis found in Blood Type B individuals is not as easy to characterize as that found in Blood Type O (grain lectins -> immune provocation) or in Type A (animal proteins -> vascular permeability and tissue inflammation). Rather, Blood Type B may have developed evolutionary adaptations that makes it on the whole somewhat more resistant to the very aggressive forms of inflammation and arthritis.

Blood Type B (and AB, who has the B antigen as well) appears to have a unique sensitivity to a class of agglutinins called galectins. Galectins are found in all animals, but most notably in chicken meat. Galectins are considered a type of internal lectin made by higher animals and used for a variety of specialized functions, especially within the liver. They bind several different galactose-antigens, and that is probably the reason that chicken seems to agglutinate the cells of Blood Types B and AB. Several galectins are known to involve themselves in the inflammatory process—another good reason to avoid chicken if you are Blood Type B or AB.

Blood Type B is especially susceptible to autoimmune diseases that develop as a result of slow-growing viruses and infections. These include rheumatoid arthritis, lupus, and scleroderma. For example, urinary tract infections, to which Blood Type B individuals are prone, are known triggers for subsequent inflammatory diseases. Simply put, when the immune system launches an attack on the infectious agent, it tends to overreact, causing inflammation.

Blood Type B might also have a special risk for inflammatory heart conditions, such as rheumatic heart disease. Factor VIII, one of the important blood-clotting factors, and itself somewhat of a promoter of inflammation, is typically elevated in Blood Type A. However, during the acute stage of inflammation, it is elevated instead in Blood Type B.

In addition, Blood Type B is highly susceptible to the inflammatory effects of lectins in some common grains, most notably wheat and corn. The lectins exacerbate the tendency for hyperimmunity, which is characteristic of autoimmune diseases.

Secretors and Non-Secretors

ALTHOUGH EVERYONE CARRIES a blood type antigen on their blood cells, about 80 percent of the population also secretes blood type antigens into body fluids, such as saliva, mucus, and sperm. These people are called secretors. The 20 percent of the population that does not secrete blood type antigens into body fluids are called non-secretors. Being a secretor is independent of your ABO type. Thus there are both Blood Type O secretors and Blood Type O non-secretors.

Since blood type antigens are crucial to immune defense, being unable to secrete them into body fluids can place non-secretors at a disadvantage. In general, non-secretors are far more likely to suffer from immune diseases than secretors, especially when the disease is provoked by an infectious organism. Non-secretors also have genetically induced difficulties removing immune complexes from their tissues, provoking inflammatory conditions.

Research has shown the following about non-secretors:

- Non-secretors are more prone to generalized inflammation than secretors.
- Non-secretors account for 80 percent of all fibromyalgia sufferers, irrespective of blood type.
- Non-secretors have an increased prevalence of a variety of autoimmune diseases, including ankylosing spondylitis, reactive arthritis, psoriatic arthritis, Sjögren's syndrome, multiple sclerosis, and Graves' disease. For example, although non-secretors make up only about 20 percent of the population, they account for nearly 50 percent of all cases of ankylosing spondylitis.
- Non-secretors have an elevated risk for recurrent urinary tract infections, and between 55 and 60 percent of non-secretors have been found to develop renal scars even with the regular use of antibiotic treatment for UTIs.

Since secretor status is a critical factor in preventing and treating arthritis, the individualized Blood Type Diet plans include variations based on secretor status. See Appendix C for information about secretor status testing.

FOR MORE INFORMATION about health factors associated with your secretor status, refer to *Live Right 4 Your Type* and the *Eat Right 4 Your Type Complete Blood Type Encyclopedia*. Extensive study references related to the blood type specificities of inflammatory disease are available for review on our Web site (www.dadamo.com).

THREE

Fighting Arthritis with Conventional and Blood Type Therapies

ARTHRITIS IS A WILY ENEMY, CAPABLE OF TAKING ON MANY forms. Symptoms may develop over time, but many of my patients report that they appear suddenly and without warning. The resulting pain, loss of function, and overall disability can be devastating, and those afflicted face a confusing array of options for treatment.

Nutritional strategies, which are the foundation of the Blood Type Diet, are still relatively uncommon in conventional medicine. Yet, in more than two decades treating patients with arthritis, I have seen remarkable and satisfying results using dietary adjustments.

Most of my patients fight disease using the best that conventional medicine has to offer, along with the added benefits of a diet that is genetically suited to their blood type. I advise you to do the same, educating yourself about the potential benefits and potential complications associated with various protocols.

Conventional Treatments: Pros and Cons

THE MAJOR PROBLEM with conventional medical protocols for arthritis is that they focus almost entirely on relief of symptoms. Virtually all current research is devoted to drug development. Treating arthritis and related conditions is big business, but relatively little attention is given to underlying causes and prevention.

Common treatments being used for arthritis include the following:

Over-the-counter analgesics, such as Tylenol, offer mild pain relief and fever reduction. They are not anti-inflammatories.

Non-steroidal anti-inflammatory drugs (NSAIDs), such as ibuprofen, have long been used to reduce arthritis pain and decrease inflammation. However, gastrointestinal complications, and even ulcers, are common side effects of NSAIDS. Three new drugs, introduced in the 1990s (Celebrex®, Vioxx® and Bextra®) have been heavily promoted as causing fewer ulcers and other gastrointestinal complications than older anti-inflammatory medicines. In addition, they inhibit an enzyme called COX-2, which triggers inflammation, while sparing an enzyme called COX-1, which helps protect the stomach lining. But the safety of these drugs has been called into question recently. A new study, focused on arthritis patients at high risk of recurrent ulcers, shows that Celebrex did not offer the level of protection previously claimed; nearly 10 percent of patients would develop another bleeding ulcer each year. Of the study patients receiving Celebrex, about 5 percent had recurrent bleeding during the six months of research, compared with about 6.5 percent for older medications, such as Prilosec. In addition, the newer anti-inflammatory drugs did not protect as many patients from dangerous kidney complications as past studies showed.

Blood Type O individuals should be wary of using NSAIDs and should look for natural alternatives when possible.

Corticosteroids are powerful anti-inflammatory hormones made naturally in the body or produced synthetically. Corticosteroids are used to treat many autoimmune inflammatory conditions because they decrease inflammation and suppress the immune system. Corticosteroids can be given by mouth, in creams applied to the skin, or by injection. Short-term side effects of corticosteroids include swelling, increased appetite, weight gain, and mood swings. These side effects generally stop when the drug is stopped. It can be dangerous to stop taking corticosteroids suddenly, so it is very important that the doctor and patient work together when changing the corticosteroid dose. Side effects that may occur after long-term use of corticosteroids include stretch marks, excessive hair growth, osteoporosis, high blood pressure, damage to the arteries, high blood sugar, infections, and cataracts. Because of the link between Blood Type A and high levels of cortisol during stress, Blood Type A individuals should minimize the use of corticosteroids when possible—especially if there are sleep disturbances.

Viscosupplements replace hyaluronic acid (HA), a substance that helps lubricate the joints, which is lost in patients with osteoarthritis. They are approved by the U.S. Food and Drug Administration for the treatment of knee pain in osteoarthritis patients who are unresponsive to nonpharmacologic measures and analgesic medications and who have experienced significantly increased flares of inflammation or extensive inflammation in one or a few joints. Two drugs, Hyalgan (hyaluronan) and Synvisc (hylan), are injected directly into the joint to replace the hyaluronic acid and help the joint move freely. Researchers are currently testing whether hyaluronic acid can slow the progression of osteoarthritis.

Enbrel (etanercept) is a genetically engineered protein that helps reduce symptoms and inhibits the progression of structural damage in adult patients with moderate to severe rheumatoid arthritis who have not responded well to other treatments. Enbrel works by binding to and inactivating a compound called tumor necrosis factor that is involved in the cascade of chemical reactions that cause inflammation.

The usual side effects are injection site reactions that include redness, itching, bruising, or pain at the injection site, upper respiratory infections, allergic reactions, stuffy nose, cough, sore throat, poor wound healing, upset stomach, and headache. There have been very rare reports of serious nervous system disorders such as multiple sclerosis, seizures or inflammation of the nerves of the eyes, and serious infections, including sepsis and tuberculosis.

Surgery may be required to repair damage to a joint after injury or to restore function or relieve pain in a joint damaged by arthritis. The doctor may recommend arthroscopic surgery, bone fusion, or arthroplasty (also known as total joint replacement, in which the damaged joint is removed and replaced with an artificial one).

Arthroscopic knee surgery is performed on more than 300,000 Americans each year who suffer from osteoarthritis to clear out debris or repair damaged cartilage. It, too, is coming under harsh scrutiny. Recent government research suggests that this surgery may be worthless. A provocative study compared arthroscopic knee surgery for osteoarthritis to a sham procedure and found no difference in the outcomes. In a type of study only rarely conducted, some patients got a real knee operation, while others underwent the sham surgery. At every point over the next two years, those who had the fake surgery could climb stairs and walk slightly faster on average than those who had had real operations. The study authors stated that the benefits derived seemed to come from a placebo effect, not the surgery itself.

BEFORE BEGINNING any treatment plan involving medications, injections, or surgery, make sure you thoroughly discuss all of the pros and cons with your physician. Understand the full implications of each therapy and assess it in the context of your personal medical history, the severity of your condition, and your risk factors for digestive problems, immune deficiencies, or metabolic imbalances.

Fighting Arthritis with the Blood Type Diet

THE BLOOD TYPE DIET is designed to work in a complementary way with other therapies. If you are being treated for an arthritic condition, talk to your physician before beginning this program and keep him or her informed of your progress. Never stop taking medication without consulting your doctor, even if you think you no longer need it. It can be dangerous to abruptly cease certain medications.

The Blood Type Diet and its associated strategies can benefit you by:

Attacking the underlying cause of arthritis. The Blood Type Diet promotes a healthy immune system, reducing the potential for infections that can trigger arthritis and normalizing the inflammatory response.

Relieving the symptoms of arthritis. Arthritis patients using the Blood Type Diet typically experience a reduction of pain and inflammation. Supported by the exercise and lifestyle guidelines, they also report more energy and greater joint flexibility.

Counterbalancing the side effects of conventional treatments. Most medical treatments for arthritis have side effects, some of which are severe. When used in conjunction with NSAIDs, for example, the Blood Type Diet can help minimize gastrointestinal problems. When used in conjunction with corticosteroid treatment, the Blood Type Diet can help you avoid or minimize weight gain, edema, and depression.

Minimizing the risk of medical complications related to arthritis. Arthritic conditions do not exist in a vacuum. Scientists are increasingly discovering correlations between the inflammatory properties of arthritis and the risk for other serious diseases, including heart disease, kidney disease, and depression. By recognizing and addressing the blood type–specific risk factors for these diseases, you can help prevent their occurrence.

Establishing overall health and fitness. The arthritis blood type plan utilizes the best of naturopathic medicine, combined with individualized diet, exercise, and lifestyle strategies that support maximum health. The Blood Type Diet is nutritionally tailored to emphasize foods that support digestive, immune, and metabolic balance. It fights obesity (a factor in the development of osteoarthritis) and improves strength and fitness by reducing fat and building lean muscle mass.

ARE YOU READY to start? Find your blood type section, and we'll get you on the right diet for your type to fight arthritis.

PART II

Individualized Blood Type Plans

Blood Type

O

BLOOD TYPE O DIET OUTCOME: CURED IN THREE DAYS
"I was cured from arthritis in three days of being on the diet and even when I cheat from time to time I still feel great! Thank you for all the wonderful info. I tell everyone about this life change and what it has done for me."*

BLOOD TYPE O DIET OUTCOME: MOVEMENT RESTORED
"The Blood Type Diet has given me back my quality of life. I was getting terrible headaches that lasted from two to five days. I had trouble with arthritis and was getting nowhere with my aerobics workouts, as I would need to quit after ten minutes. I was beginning to think I would need to give up most aspects of my favorite hobbies, which involve work with my dogs."

BLOOD TYPE O DIET OUTCOME: PAIN-FREE AT LAST
"I was diagnosed with chronic non-specific seronegative inflammatory arthritis (possibly psoriatic arthritis). The Blood Type Diet, particularly wheat, corn, and oat avoidance, has led to decreased pain and inflammation. Returning to a wheat-based diet for even one day causes an arthritic flare-up."

*Self-reported outcomes from the Blood Type Diet web site, www.dadamo.com

BLOOD TYPE O HAS A GENERALLY HARDY IMMUNE SYSTEM but a tendency to hyperimmunity and accompanying inflammation. Inflammatory diseases, such as rheumatoid arthritis and fibromyalgia, are more common in Blood Type O individuals than in the other blood types. Inflammatory bowel diseases such as Crohn's disease and ulcerative colitis, commonly associated with arthritis, disproportionately afflict Blood Type O individuals.

Blood Type O's vulnerability to a range of inflammatory problems is related to having the greatest levels and variety of anti-blood type antibodies. This is heightened by the presence of certain lectins in the diet that are O-reactive. Chief among these is the wheat germ lectin, which is not O-specific but which always reacts more negatively in Blood Type O individuals. Perhaps this is because Type O has higher levels of the binding sugar (NAG) for wheat lectin in its digestive mucous than the other blood types. Time and again I've seen remarkable improvements in my Blood Type O patients who suffer from arthritis, fibromyalgia, and other inflammatory conditions when they eliminate wheat and corn from their diets.

Other grain lectins can also impair musculoskeletal integrity in Blood Type O. The effects of corn lectin on Blood Type O bone structure can be observed anthropologically. Ancient Native Americans, almost exclusively Blood Type O, were hunter-gatherers. Based upon anthropological studies of bone remains, it is possible to trace the exact period when corn was introduced into these cultures. Prior to corn becoming a staple, the bones show little arthritis or thinning. After corn was introduced, bone deformation began, including major changes to the teeth structure and jaw (periodontal disease).

Blood Type O has a high degree of reactivity with the lectin found in the common lentil bean (*Lens culinaris*), producing inflammatory conditions. Research has demonstrated that a very good experimental model of human rheumatoid arthritis can be produced in laboratory rabbits by injecting their joints with the lentil lectin.

Gastrointestinal health is a key to Blood Type O's arthritis-fighting strategy. Over one-third of our entire immune system is located in the gastrointestinal tract, and it is commonly accepted that gut inflammation is associated with joint inflammation. Blood Type O's strong association with gastrointestinal diseases is highly relevant to any discussion of arthritis. For example, research has demonstrated a strong connection between *H. pylori* infection and arthritis. *H. pylori* infection, which is responsible for most cases of ulcers, is highly specific to the fucose sugar of Blood Type O.

The bottom line: Blood Type O can effectively fight arthritis by eating the right diet for your type.

Blood Type O Arthritis-Fighting Food Analysis

ANTI-INFLAMMATORY FOODS	PRO-INFLAMMATORY FOODS
Lean, organic, grass-fed red meat	Wheat and wheat by-products
Richly oiled cold-water fish	Corn and corn by-products
Flax (linseed) oil	Cow's milk–based dairy foods
Olive oil	Corn, cottonseed, peanut, safflower oil
Seaweeds	Lentil beans
Onion	White potatoes
Sweet potato	Bell peppers
Spinach, kale, collards	Eggplant
Pineapple	Tomato and tomato products
Blueberries, cherries, elderberries	Kiwi, oranges, tangerines
Ginger	Food additives
Cayenne pepper	Processed sugar
Turmeric	Coffee (caffeinated/ decaffeinated)
Green tea	

The Mind/Body Factor

SOME AUTOIMMUNE INFLAMMATORY DISEASES, such as fibromyalgia, are believed to be related to abnormalities in the neuroendocrine system—in particular, the regulation of noradrenaline and dopamine. For this reason, many people with these conditions suffer from depression. This finding has special relevance for Blood Type O individuals. Because of a link between the blood type gene and the dopamine beta hydroxylase gene, Blood Type O tends to have a harder time regulating dopamine, a chemical intimately connected to the activity of the satiety, or pleasure, centers of the brain. This imbalance is a possible explanation for Blood Type O's general susceptibility to manic-depressive illness. Now we see a further connection with certain inflammatory diseases to which Blood Type O is also susceptible. The bottom line: Blood Type O individuals with arthritis may be more inclined to suffer from depression.

A Word to the Wise Type O: Glucosamine and Chondroitin

MANY OF MY PATIENTS have wanted to know if they should take glucosamine and chondroitin. Blood Type O can benefit from taking glucosamine but should avoid chondroitin. Here's why: Glucosamine helps to block inflammation-producing lectins, especially wheat germ lectin, by acting as a decoy. The lectin binds to it instead of binding to your intestinal lining. However, you may want to choose your form of glucosamine carefully; try to find the acetylated form (N-acetyl glucosamine, or NAG) and preferably use that instead of the sulfated form (glucosamine sulfate).

Chondroitin is a different matter. If we were to analyze the structure of chondroitin, we would see that it is composed of a repeating sugar, N-acetyl galactosamine. N-acetyl galactosamine is the Blood Type A antigen. Thus, by consuming large amounts of chondroitin, Blood Type O is essentially provoking its immune system with what amounts to an incompatible blood transfusion. Forget about chondroitin; just use the glucosamine.

A good herbal choice for arthritis Blood Type Os derives from the frankincense bush (*Boswellia serulata*). Boswellia contains boswellic acids, which have been shown to have an anti-inflammatory action—much like the conventional nonsteroidal anti-inflammatory drugs

(NSAIDs) used to treat inflammatory conditions. Boswellia inhibits pro-inflammatory mediators in the body, such as leukotrienes.

In the ancient Ayurvedic medical texts of India, the gummy exudate from boswellia is grouped with other gum resins and referred to collectively as guggals. Historically, the guggals were recommended by Ayurvedic physicians for a variety of conditions, including osteoarthritis, rheumatoid arthritis, diarrhea, dysentery, pulmonary disease, and ringworm.

Blood Type O: The Foods

THE BLOOD TYPE O Arthritis Diet is specifically adapted for the prevention and management of arthritis. A new category, **Super Beneficial**, highlights powerful arthritis-fighting foods for Blood Type O. The **Neutral** category has also been adjusted to de-emphasize foods that are less advantageous for you. Foods designated **Neutral: Allowed Infrequently** should be minimized or avoided entirely.

Your secretor status can influence your ability to fully digest and metabolize certain foods, so various adjustments in the values are made for non-secretors. If you do not know your secretor type, the odds are that you can safely use the "secretor" values, since the majority of the

Food Values

SUPER BENEFICIAL	Foods that are known to have specific disease-fighting qualities for your blood type.
BENEFICIAL	Foods with components that enhance the metabolic, immune, or structural health of you blood type.
NEUTRAL: Allowed Infrequently	Foods that normally have no direct type effect but may impede your progress when consumed regularly.
AVOID	Foods with components that are harmful to your blood type.

population (approximately 80 percent) are secretors. However, I urge you to get tested, since the variations are important for non-secretors who want to maximize the effectiveness of the Blood Type Diet.

The food charts are divided into three sections. The top of the chart suggests the average portion size and quantity per week or day, according to secretor status. These recommendations do *not* apply to the category **Neutral: Allowed Infrequently;** those foods should be eaten rarely, if at all. The charts also indicate differences in frequency for some foods, based on ethnic heritage. It has been my experience that this factor has an impact upon the individual's ability to fully digest certain foods. For the purposes of blood type food choices, persons of Hispanic heritage should follow the recommendations for Caucasians, and North American Native peoples should follow the recommendations for Asians.

The middle section of the chart gives the food values. The bottom section lists variants based on secretor status.

For your convenience, we have included a number of product names (Ezekiel bread, Worcestershire sauce, etc.). However, keep in mind that commercial formulations vary among brands and regions. Even though a product may be listed as acceptable for you, always check its ingredients; do not use products that contain **Avoid** ingredients for your blood type. Of course, you may choose to make your own version of commercial products, such as bread and mayonnaise, using ingredients that suit your blood type. There are hundreds of delicious recipes for every blood type available on our Web site (www.dadamo.com) and in the book *Cook Right 4 Your Type: The Practical Kitchen Companion to* Eat Right 4 Your Type.

Meat/Poultry

Protein, in the form of lean, organic meat, is critical for Blood Type O and is the key to digestive, immune, and metabolic health. This is even more important for non-secretors. Blood Type O thrives on a high-protein diet, necessary to build lean muscle mass, which in turn minimizes the risk of joint deterioration. High-quality animal protein is easily digested by Blood Type O, essential for digestive health and avoidance of the gut inflammation that can trigger arthritic conditions.

Limit organ meats if you have gout. They are sources of purine, which is known to exacerbate that condition.

Choose only the best-quality (preferably free-range), chemical-, antibiotic-, and pesticide-free, low-fat meats and poultry. Grass-fed cattle and buffalo are far superior to grain-fed.

BLOOD TYPE O: MEAT/POULTRY			
Portion: 4–6 oz (men); 2–5 oz (women and children)			
	African	Caucasian	Asian
Secretor	6–9	6–9	6–9
Non-Secretor	7–12	7–12	7–11
		Times per week	

SUPER BENEFICIAL	BENEFICIAL	NEUTRAL: Allowed Frequently	NEUTRAL: Allowed Infrequently	AVOID
Beef	Heart (calf)	Chicken		All commercially processed meats
Buffalo	Liver (calf)	Cornish hen		Bacon/Ham/Pork
Lamb	Mutton	Duck		Quail
	Sweetbreads	Goat		Turtle
	Veal	Goose		
	Venison	Grouse		
		Guinea hen		
		Horse		
		Ostrich		
		Partridge		
		Pheasant		
		Rabbit		
		Squab		
		Squirrel		
		Turkey		

Special Variants: *Non-Secretor* BENEFICIAL: ostrich, partridge, pheasant, rabbit, squab; NEUTRAL (Allowed Frequently): lamb, liver (calf), quail, turtle.

Fish/Seafood

Fish and seafood represent a secondary source of high-quality protein for Blood Type O. In particular, richly oiled cold-water fish like cod, halibut, red snapper, and trout are SUPER BENEFICIAL for Type O. These fish contain beneficial omega-3 fatty acids, such as docosahexaenoic acid (DHA) and eicosapentaenoic acid (EPA) and are considered anti-inflammatory; they reduce the effects of pro-inflammatory fats.

BLOOD TYPE O: FISH/SEAFOOD			
Portion: 4–6 oz (men); 2–5 oz (women and children)			
	African	Caucasian	Asian
Secretor	2–4	3–5	2–5
Non-Secretor	2–5	4–5	4–5
			Times per week

SUPER BENEFICIAL	BENEFICIAL	NEUTRAL: Allowed Frequently	NEUTRAL: Allowed Infrequently	AVOID
Cod	Bass (all)	Beluga	Anchovy	Abalone
Halibut	Perch (all)	Bluefish	Clam	Barracuda
Red snapper	Pike	Bullhead	Crab	Catfish
Trout (rainbow)	Shad	Butterfish	Lobster	Conch
	Sole (except gray)	Carp	Mussel	Frog
	Sturgeon	Caviar (sturgeon)		Herring (pickled/ smoked)
	Swordfish	Chub		Muskel-lunge
	Tilefish	Croaker		Octopus
	Yellowtail	Cusk		Pollock
		Drum		Salmon (smoked)
		Eel		Salmon roe
		Flounder		Squid (calamari)
		Gray sole		
		Grouper		
		Haddock		
		Hake		

SUPER BENEFICIAL	BENEFICIAL	NEUTRAL: Allowed Frequently	NEUTRAL: Allowed Infrequently	AVOID
		Halfmoon fish		
		Harvest fish		
		Herring (fresh)		
		Mackerel		
		Mahi-mahi		
		Monkfish		
		Mullet		
		Opaleye fish		
		Orange roughy		
		Oysters		
		Parrot fish		
		Pickerel		
		Pompano		
		Porgy		
		Rosefish		
		Sailfish		
		Salmon		
		Sardine		
		Scallops		
		Scrod		
		Shark		
		Shrimp		
		Smelt		
		Snail (*Helix pomatia*/ escargot)		
		Sucker		
		Sunfish		
		Tilapia		

SUPER BENEFICIAL	BENEFICIAL	NEUTRAL: Allowed Frequently	NEUTRAL: Allowed Infrequently	AVOID
		Trout (brook/ sea)		
		Tuna		
		Turtle		
		Weakfish		
		Whitefish		
		Whiting		

Special Variants: *Non-Secretor* BENEFICIAL: hake, herring (fresh), mackerel, sardine; NEUTRAL (Allowed Frequently): bass, catfish, halibut, red snapper, salmon roe; AVOID: anchovy, crab, mussel.

Dairy/Eggs

Most dairy foods should be avoided by Blood Type O, especially if you have arthritis. They are extremely pro-inflammatory for Type O. Eggs can be consumed in moderation. They are a good source of omega-3 docosahexaenoic acid (DHA) and can help build active tissue mass. Ghee (clarified butter) is a good source of butyrate, which supports intestinal health. Do your best to find eggs and dairy products that meet organic standards.

BLOOD TYPE O: EGGS			
Portion: 1 egg			
	African	Caucasian	Asian
Secretor	1–4	3–6	3–4
Non-Secretor	2–5	3–6	3–4
	Times per week		

BLOOD TYPE O: MILK AND YOGURT

Portion: 4–6 oz (men); 2–5 oz (women and children)

	African	Caucasian	Asian
Secretor	0–1	0–3	0–2
Non-Secretor	0	0–2	0–3
	Times per week		

BLOOD TYPE O: CHEESE

Portion: 3 oz (men); 2 oz (women and children)

	African	Caucasian	Asian
Secretor	0–1	0–2	0–1
Non-Secretor	0	0–1	0
	Times per week		

SUPER BENEFICIAL	BENEFICIAL	NEUTRAL: Allowed Frequently	NEUTRAL: Allowed Infrequently	AVOID
	Ghee (clarified butter)	Egg (chicken/ duck)	Butter	American cheese
			Farmer cheese	Blue cheese
			Feta	Brie
			Goat cheese	Buttermilk
			Mozzarella	Camembert
				Casein
				Cheddar
				Colby
				Cottage cheese
				Cream cheese
				Edam
				Egg (goose/ quail)
				Emmenthal
				Gouda

SUPER BENEFICIAL	BENEFICIAL	NEUTRAL: Allowed Frequently	NEUTRAL: Allowed Infrequently	AVOID
				Gruyère
				Half-and-half
				Ice cream
				Jarlsberg
				Kefir
				Milk (cow/goat)
				Monterey Jack
				Muenster
				Neufchâtel
				Paneer
				Parmesan
				Provolone
				Quark
				Ricotta
				Sherbet
				Sour cream
				Swiss cheese
				Whey
				Yogurt

Special Variants: *Non-Secretor* NEUTRAL (Allowed Frequently): Egg (goose/quail); AVOID: farmer cheese, feta, goat cheese, mozzarella.

Oils

Olive oil, a monounsaturated oil, is SUPER BENEFICIAL for Blood Type O. Constituents in olive oil, such as flavonoids, squalenes, and polyphenols, act as powerful antioxidants. Use it as your primary cooking oil. Also SUPER BENEFICIAL is flax oil (linseed), high in alpha-linolenic acid (ALA), which has anti-inflammatory properties. Be aware that some oils are high in omega-6 fatty acids, which can stimulate the inflammatory response. These include corn, cottonseed, peanut, and safflower oils. Secretors have a bit of an edge in digesting oils over non-secretors and probably benefit a bit more from their consumption.

BLOOD TYPE O: OILS			
Portion: 1 tblsp			
	African	Caucasian	Asian
Secretor	3–8	4–8	5–8
Non-Secretor	1–7	3–5	3–6
	Times per week		

SUPER BENEFICIAL	BENEFICIAL	NEUTRAL: Allowed Frequently	NEUTRAL: Allowed Infrequently	AVOID
Flax (linseed) Olive		Almond Black currant seed Sesame Walnut	Borage seed Canola Cod liver	Avocado Castor Coconut Corn Cottonseed Evening primrose Peanut Safflower Soy Sunflower Wheat germ

Special Variants: *Non-Secretor* BENEFICIAL: almond, walnut; NEUTRAL (Allowed Frequently): coconut, flax (linseed); AVOID: borage, canola, cod liver.

Nuts and Seeds

Raw flaxseeds (linseeds) are helpful for a strong immune system, providing beneficial omega-3 fatty acids. Walnuts are also SUPER BENEFICIAL. They are one of the best plant sources of omega-3 fatty acids. Walnuts are also highly effective in inhibiting gastrointestinal toxicity.

Many nuts and seeds, including beechnut, sunflower seeds, and chestnuts, possess lectin or other immune reactivity for Blood Type O.

BLOOD TYPE O: NUTS AND SEEDS			
Portion: Whole (handful); Nut Butters (2 tblsp)			
	African	Caucasian	Asian
Secretor	2–5	2–5	2–4
Non-Secretor	5–7	5–7	5–7
		Times per week	

SUPER BENEFICIAL	BENEFICIAL	NEUTRAL: Allowed Frequently	NEUTRAL: Allowed Infrequently	AVOID
Flax (linseed) Walnut	Pumpkin seed	Almond Butternut Filbert (hazelnut) Hickory Macadamia Pecan Pignolia (pine nut)	Almond butter Almond cheese Almond milk Safflower seed Sesame butter (tahini) Sesame seed	Beechnut Brazil nut Cashew Chestnut Litchi Peanut Peanut butter Pistachio Poppy seed Sunflower butter Sunflower seed

Special Variants: *Non-Secretor* NEUTRAL (Allowed Frequently): flax (linseed); AVOID: almond cheese, almond milk, safflower seed.

Beans and Legumes

Essentially carnivores when it comes to protein requirements, Blood Type Os should minimize consumption of beans and legumes. Many of them, such as lentils, contain pro-inflammatory lectins. Given the choice, get your protein from animal foods.

BLOOD TYPE O: BEANS AND LEGUMES			
Portion: 1 cup (cooked)			
	African	Caucasian	Asian
Secretor	1–3	1–3	2–4
Non-Secretor	0–2	0–3	2–4
	Times per week		

SUPER BENEFICIAL	BENEFICIAL	NEUTRAL: Allowed Frequently	NEUTRAL: Allowed Infrequently	AVOID
Fava (broad) bean	Adzuki bean Black-eyed pea	Bean (green/ snap/ string) Black bean Cannellini bean Jicama bean Lima bean Miso Mung bean/ sprout Northern bean	Garbanzo (chickpea)	Copper bean Kidney bean Lentil (all) Navy bean Pinto bean Tamarind bean

SUPER BENEFICIAL	BENEFICIAL	NEUTRAL: Allowed Frequently	NEUTRAL: Allowed Infrequently	AVOID
		Pea (green/ pod/ snow) Soy bean Soy cheese Soy milk Tempeh Tofu White bean		

Special Variants: *Non-Secretor* NEUTRAL (Allowed Frequently): adzuki bean, black-eyed pea; AVOID: fava (broad) bean, garbanzo (chickpea), soy (all).

Grains and Starches

Blood Type O does poorly on corn, wheat, sorghum, barley, and many of their by-products (sweeteners, etc.). Wheat is a leading factor in the development of inflammatory conditions for Blood Type O—especially arthritis, fibromyalgia, and inflammatory bowel disease. Non-secretors have even greater wheat sensitivity. Non-secretors should avoid oats as well.

BLOOD TYPE O: GRAINS AND STARCHES			
Portion: ½ cup dry (grains or pastas); 1 muffin; 2 slices of bread			
	African	Caucasian	Asian
Secretor	1–6	1–6	1–6
Non-Secretor	0–3	0–3	0–3
		Times per week	

SUPER BENEFICIAL	BENEFICIAL	NEUTRAL: Allowed Frequently	NEUTRAL: Allowed Infrequently	AVOID
	Essene bread (manna)	Amaranth	Buckwheat	Barley
		Ezekiel bread	Millet	Cornmeal
		Kamut	Oat bran	Couscous
		Quinoa	Oat flour	Grits
		Soy flour/ products	Oatmeal	Popcorn
		Spelt (whole)	Rice (whole)	Sorghum
		Spelt flour/ products	Rice bran	Wheat (re-fined/un-bleached)
		100% sprouted grain products (except Essene)	Rice cake	Wheat (semolina)
			Rice flour	Wheat (white flour)
			Rice milk	Wheat bran
			Rice (wild)	Wheat germ
			Rye (whole)	Wheat (whole)
			Rye flour/ products	
			Soba noodles (100% buck-wheat)	
			Tapioca	
			Teff	

Special Variants: *Non-Secretor* AVOID: buckwheat, oat flour, soba noodles (100% buckwheat), soy flour/products, spelt (whole), spelt flour/products, tapioca.

Vegetables

Vegetables provide a rich source of antioxidants and fiber, and the right choices can help Blood Type O balance immune functions. Fucose-containing seaweeds are SUPER BENEFICIAL in blocking lectin activity, and serve as a food source for friendly colon bacteria, thus reducing gut inflammation. Onions are high in quercetin, a flavonoid with potent anti-inflammatory properties. Sweet potatoes are rich in vitamins A and B_6, which stabilize immune function. Several vegetables are pro-inflammatory for Blood Type O and should be minimized or avoided. These include the so-called nightshade family—white potatoes, bell peppers, eggplant, and tomatoes.

An item's value also applies to its juice, unless otherwise noted.

BLOOD TYPE O: VEGETABLES			
Portion: 1 cup, prepared (cooked or raw)			
	African	Caucasian	Asian
Secretor Super/ Beneficials	Unlimited	Unlimited	Unlimited
Secretor Neutrals	2–5	2–5	2–5
Non-Secretor Super/Beneficials	Unlimited	Unlimited	Unlimited
Non-Secretor Neutrals	2–3	2–3	2–3
	Times per day		

SUPER BENEFICIAL	BENEFICIAL	NEUTRAL: Allowed Frequently	NEUTRAL: Allowed Infrequently	AVOID
Broccoli	Artichoke	Arugula	Brussels sprouts	Alfalfa sprouts
Collards	Beet greens	Asparagus	Cabbage	Aloe
Garlic	Chicory	Asparagus pea	Eggplant	Cauliflower
Kale	Escarole	Bamboo shoot	Olive (Greek/ green/ Spanish)	Corn
Onion (all)	Horse-radish	Beet	Peppers (all)	Cucumber
Potato (sweet)	Kohlrabi	Bok choy	Tomato	Leek
Seaweeds	Lettuce (Romaine)	Carrot	Yam	Mushroom (shiitake/ silver dollar)
Spinach	Mushroom (abalone/ enoki/ maitake/ oyster/ porto-bello/ straw/ tree ear)	Celeriac		Mustard greens
		Celery		Olive (black)
		Daikon radish		Pickles (in brine or vinegar)
		Dandelion		Potato
		Endive		
		Fennel		
		Fiddlehead fern		

SUPER BENEFICIAL	BENEFICIAL	NEUTRAL: Allowed Frequently	NEUTRAL: Allowed Infrequently	AVOID
	Okra Parsnip Pumpkin Swiss chard Turnip	Lettuce (except Romaine) Poi Radicchio Radish/ sprouts Rappini (broccoli rabe) Rutabaga Scallion Shallot Squash Water chestnut Watercress Zucchini		Rhubarb

Special Variants: *Non-Secretor* BENEFICIAL: carrot, fiddlehead fern; NEUTRAL (Allowed Frequently): lettuce (Romaine), mushroom (silver dollar), parsnip, turnip; AVOID: Brussels sprouts, cabbage, eggplant, olive (all), poi.

Fruits and Fruit Juices

Fruits are rich in antioxidants and many, such as blueberries, elderberries, and cherries, are high in anthocyanins, which enhance collagen integrity. Collagen is essential for bone and connective tissue health. Pineapple contains bromelain, a powerful enzyme that has an anti-inflammatory effect on muscle and tissue. Several fruits, such as kiwi and oranges, contain Blood Type O–reactive lectins, and these should be avoided.

An item's value also applies to its juice, unless otherwise noted.

BLOOD TYPE O: FRUITS AND FRUIT JUICES			
Portion: 1 cup			
	African	Caucasian	Asian
Secretor	2–4	3–5	3–5
Non-Secretor	1–3	1–3	1–3
			Times per day

SUPER BENEFICIAL	BENEFICIAL	NEUTRAL: Allowed Frequently	NEUTRAL: Allowed Infrequently	AVOID
Blueberry	Banana	Apple	Apricot	Asian pear
Cherry (all)	Fig (fresh/ dried)	Boysenberry	Currant	Avocado
Iderberry (dark blue/ purple)	Guava	Breadfruit	Date	Bitter melon
Pineapple	Mango	Canang melon	Quince	Blackberry
	Plum (all)	Casaba melon	Raisin	Cantaloupe
	Pomegranate	Christmas melon	Star fruit (carambola)	Coconut
	Prune	Cranberry	Strawberry	Honeydew melon
		Crenshaw melon		Kiwi
		Dewberry		Orange
				Plantain
				Tangerine

SUPER BENEFICIAL	BENEFICIAL	NEUTRAL: Allowed Frequently	NEUTRAL: Allowed Infrequently	AVOID
		Gooseberry		
		Grape (all)		
		Grapefruit		
		Kumquat		
		Lemon		
		Lime		
		Loganberry		
		Mulberry		
		Muskmelon		
		Nectarine		
		Papaya		
		Peach		
		Pear		
		Persian melon		
		Persimmon		
		Prickly pear		
		Raspberry		
		Sago palm		
		Spanish melon		
		Watermelon		
		Youngberry		

Special Variants: *Non-Secretor* BENEFICIAL: avocado, prickly pear; AVOID: apple, apricot, date, strawberry.

Spices/Condiments/Sweeteners

Many spices are known to have anti-inflammatory properties. The common cooking spices—rosemary, thyme, and oregano—are powerful antioxidants that exert anti-inflammatory effects. Turmeric and garlic are also anti-inflammatory. The burning substance in cayenne pepper (capsaicin) is the primary ingredient of some pain-reducing arthritis creams. Ginger inhibits the production of COX-2, an enzyme that triggers the inflammatory response. Parsley contains quercetin, which is anti-inflammatory. Many common food additives, such as guar gum and carrageenan, enhance the effects of lectins found in other foods and should be avoided. Avoid yeast if you have gout.

Use caution when using prepared condiments. Many of them contain wheat, which is a primary factor in the development of arthritis and other inflammatory conditions for Blood Type O.

SUPER BENEFICIAL	BENEFICIAL	NEUTRAL: Allowed Frequently	NEUTRAL: Allowed Infrequently	AVOID
Garlic	Carob	Agar	Arrowroot	Aspartame
Ginger	Fenugreek	Allspice	Barley malt	Capers
Parsley	Horse-radish	Almond extract	Chocolate	Carrageenan
Pepper (cayenne)		Anise	Honey	Cornstarch
Oregano		Apple pectin	Ketchup	Corn syrup
Rosemary		Basil	Maple syrup	Dextrose
Thyme		Bay leaf	Molasses	Fructose
Turmeric		Bergamot	Molasses (black-strap)	Guarana
		Caraway	Rice syrup	Gums (acacia/Arabic/guar)
		Cardamom	Soy sauce	Invert sugar
		Chervil	Sucanat	Juniper
		Chili powder		Mace
		Chive		Maltodextrin
				MSG

SUPER BENEFICIAL	BENEFICIAL	NEUTRAL: Allowed Frequently	NEUTRAL: Allowed Infrequently	AVOID
		Cilantro (coriander leaf)	Sugar (brown/white)	Nutmeg
		Cinnamon	Worcestershire sauce	Pepper (black/white)
		Clove	Yeast (baker's/brewer's)	Vinegar (except apple cider)
		Coriander		
		Cream of tartar		
		Cumin		
		Dill		
		Gelatin		
		Lecithin		
		Licorice root*		
		Marjoram		
		Mayonnaise		
		Mint (all)		
		Mustard (dry)		
		Paprika		
		Pepper (peppercorn/red flakes)		
		Saffron		
		Sage		
		Savory		
		Sea salt		
		Senna		
		Stevia		
		Tamari (wheat-free)		
		Tamarind		

SUPER BENEFICIAL	BENEFICIAL	NEUTRAL: Allowed Frequently	NEUTRAL: Allowed Infrequently	AVOID
		Tarragon		
		Vanilla		
		Vegetable glycerine		
		Vinegar (apple cider)		
		Winter-green		

Special Variants: *Non-Secretor* BENEFICIAL: basil, bay leaf, licorice root*, saffron, yeast (brewer's); NEUTRAL (Allowed Frequently): carob; AVOID: barley malt, cinnamon, honey, maple syrup, mayonnaise, rice syrup, soy sauce, stevia, sucanat, sugar (brown/white), tamari (wheat-free), vanilla, vinegar (apple cider), Worcestershire sauce.

*Do not use if you have high blood pressure.

Herbal Teas

Herbal teas can provide medicinal benefits and are excellent replacements for caffeinated drinks such as coffee, cola, and black tea. Many herbal teas are anti-inflammatory for Blood Type O. These include hops, licorice, ginger, and sarsaparilla.

SUPER BENEFICIAL	BENEFICIAL	NEUTRAL: Allowed Frequently	NEUTRAL: Allowed Infrequently	AVOID
Ginger	Chickweed	Catnip	Senna	Alfalfa
Hops	Dandelion	Chamomile		Aloe
Licorice	Fenugreek	Dong quai		Burdock
Sarsaparilla	Linden	Elder		Coltsfoot
	Mulberry	Ginseng		Corn silk

SUPER BENEFICIAL	BENEFICIAL	NEUTRAL: Allowed Frequently	NEUTRAL: Allowed Infrequently	AVOID
	Peppermint	Hawthorn		Echinacea
	Rosehip	Horehound		Gentian
	Slippery elm	Mullein		Goldenseal
		Raspberry leaf		Red clover
		Skullcap		Rhubarb
		Spearmint		Shepherd's purse
		Valerian		St. John's wort
		Vervain		Strawberry leaf
		White birch		Yellow dock
		White oak bark		
		Yarrow		

Special Variants: None.

Miscellaneous Beverages

Green tea should be part of every Blood Type O's health plan. It contains polyphenols, which enhance gastrointestinal health. Avoid or limit alcohol to an occasional glass of red wine. Alcohol can exacerbate autoimmune inflammatory conditions and may be a factor in the development of some forms of arthritis, such as gout. Avoid or limit alcohol to an occasional glass of red wine. Eliminate coffee, but consume plenty of green tea. It is believed to be a preventative agent for chronic inflammatory diseases.

SUPER BENEFICIAL	BENEFICIAL	NEUTRAL: Allowed Frequently	NEUTRAL: Allowed Infrequently	AVOID
Tea (green)	Seltzer Soda (club)	Wine (red)		Beer Coffee (reg/decaf) Liquor Soda (cola/ diet/misc.) Tea, black (reg/decaf) Wine (white)

Special Variants: *Non-Secretor* BENEFICIAL: wine (red).

Supplements

THE BLOOD TYPE O DIET offers abundant quantities of important nutrients, such as protein and iron. It is important to get as many nutrients as possible from fresh foods and use supplements only to fill in the minor deficiencies in your diet. The following supplement protocols are designed for Blood Type O individuals who are suffering from arthritis or related autoimmune conditions.

Note: If you are being treated for a medical condition, consult your doctor before taking supplements.

Blood Type O: Anti-Inflammatory Protocol

Use this protocol for 12 weeks to prevent and minimize inflammatory conditions, while balancing immune function.

SUPPLEMENT	ACTION	DOSAGE
N-acetyl glucosamine	Binds inflammatory lectins	250–500 mg, 3–4 times daily, away from food
Frankincense (*Boswellia serrata*)	Has anti-inflammatory effects	500 mg, 1–2 capsules, away from food

SUPPLEMENT	ACTION	DOSAGE
Larch arabinogalactan (Larix officinalis)	Promotes digestive and intestinal health	1 tablespoon, twice daily, in juice or water
Curcumin	Anti-inflammatory	100 mg daily with meals
Quercetin	Has anti-inflammatory effects	500 mg, twice daily, away from food
Stinging nettle root (Urtica dioica)	Prevents the production of anti-self antibodies	500 mg, twice daily, away from food
Ginger root (Rhizome zingiberis)	COX-2 inhibitor; arthritis pain reliever; digestive aid	200 mg capsule before food, as a tea or compress
Bladderwrack (Fucus vesiculosus)	Blocks the activity of complement; lectin blocker	100 mg, 2–3 times daily, with food

Blood Type O: Arthritis Pain Relief Adjunct

Use this protocol for 4 weeks to reduce pain associated with joint disease.

SUPPLEMENT	ACTION	DOSAGE
Cayenne pepper (Capsicum sp.)	Arthritis pain relief	300 mg, 1–2 capsules with meals, or topically in cream
Ginger root (Rhizome zingiberis)	COX-2 inhibitor; pain reliever	200 mg capsule before meals, as a tea or compress
Bromelain (pineapple enzyme)	Has antioxidant and anti-inflammatory properties	500 mg, 1–3 capsules daily with meals, gradually decreasing dose and frequency as symptoms improve

Blood Type O: Joint Repair Adjunct

Use this protocol for 4 weeks to promote healing and improve joint integrity.

SUPPLEMENT	ACTION	DOSAGE
Horsetail (*Equisetum arvense*)	Promotes healing and facilitates calcium absorption	500 mg, twice daily
Vitamin C (rose hips or acerola cherry)	Promotes healing	250 mg, twice daily

Blood Type O: Surgery Recovery Adjunct

When surgery is scheduled, add this protocol for 2 weeks before surgery and 2 weeks after.

SUPPLEMENT	ACTION	DOSAGE
Horse chestnut (*Aesculus hippocastanum*)	Has anti-inflammatory properties	500 mg, twice daily
Rehmannia root (*Rehmannia glutinosa*)	Promotes healing; stops bleeding; provides energy	200 mg, 1 capsule daily
Bromelain	Has anti-inflammatory and wound-healing properties	500 mg, twice daily

The Exercise Component

BLOOD TYPE O BENEFITS tremendously from brisk exercise that taxes the cardiovascular and musculoskeletal systems, and this becomes particularly important if you suffer from arthritis. The best wisdom of both conventional and naturopathic medicine is that regular exercise, including aerobic activity and weight training, is essential to your arthritis-fighting strategy. It may seem counterintuitive, since arthritis makes movement difficult and often painful. However, studies consistently show that aerobic exercise can reduce joint swelling. Strength training builds muscle, helping to support and protect joints affected by arthritis. Physical exercise also promotes lean muscle mass and reduces weight, thus lightening the load on stressed joints.

Build a balanced routine of both aerobic and strength-training activities from the following chart. If you are not accustomed to exercising or your condition is severe, start slowly and do as much as you can, striving to increase your time and endurance as you gain flexibility and strength.

EXERCISE	DURATION	FREQUENCY
Aerobics	40–60 minutes	3–4 x week
Weight training	30–45 minutes	3–4 x week
Running	40–45 minutes	3–4 x week
Calisthenics	30–45 minutes	3 x week
Treadmill	30 minutes	3 x week
Kickboxing	30–45 minutes	3 x week
Cycling	30 minutes	3 x week
Contact sports	60 minutes	2–3 x week
In-line/roller skating	30 minutes	2–3 x week

3 Steps to Effective Exercise

1. Warm up with stretching and flexibility movements before you start your aerobic exercise.
2. To achieve maximum cardiovascular benefits, work toward an elevated heart rate that is about 70 percent of your capacity. Once you reach the elevated rate, continue exercising to maintain that rate for twenty to thirty minutes. To calculate your maximum heart rate and performance level:
   - Subtract your age from 220.
   - Multiply the difference by .70 (or .60 if you are over age sixty). This is the high end of your performance.
   - Multiply the remainder by .50. This is the low end of your performance.

3. Finish each aerobic session with at least a five-minute cooldown of stretching and relaxation moves.

Getting Started: The First Month

IF YOU ARE NEW to the Blood Type Diet, the following guidelines will introduce you to the Blood Type O regimen over a period of one month. Follow these recommendations as closely as possible, using a journal to record your personal experiences with the diet. In addition to factors that are measurable in laboratory tests, take the time to note changes in your energy levels, pain levels, sleep patterns, digestion, and overall well-being.

Blood Type O Arthritis Diet Checklist

Eat small to moderate portions of high-quality, lean, organic ☐ meat several times a week for strength, energy, and digestive health. Meat should be prepared medium to rare for the best health effects. If you charbroil, or cook meat well-done, use a marinade composed of beneficial ingredients, such as cherry juice, spices, and herbs.

Include regular portions of richly oiled cold-water fish. Fish ☐ oils can help counter inflammatory conditions, improve thyroid function, and balance immune activity.

Consume little or no dairy foods, which provoke inflammation ☐ for Blood Type O.

Eliminate wheat and wheat-based products from your diet. ☐ They are the primary culprits in many arthritic and autoimmune diseases.

Limit your intake of beans, as they are not a particularly good ☐ protein source for Type Os. Some contain reactive lectins that can trigger inflammation.

Eat lots of BENEFICIAL fruits and vegetables. ☐

If you need a daily dose of caffeine, replace coffee with green ☐
tea. It isn't acidic and has substantially less caffeine than a
cup of coffee.

Use BENEFICIAL and NEUTRAL nuts and dried fruits for snacks. ☐

Avoid foods that are Type O red flags, especially wheat, corn, ☐
kidney beans, navy beans, lentils, peanuts, potatoes, and
cauliflower.

Week 1

Blood Type Diet and Supplements

- Eliminate your most harmful AVOID foods—wheat and dairy. These foods
  are the primary triggers for inflammatory conditions.

- Include your most important BENEFICIAL foods on a regular schedule
  throughout the week. For example, have lean red meat 5 times, and omega-
  3–rich fish 3 to 4 times, with lots of BENEFICIAL vegetables and fruit.

- Incorporate at least 1 SUPER BENEFICIAL food into your daily diet. For
  example, eat slices of fresh pineapple or a seaweed salad.

- If you're a coffee drinker, begin to wean yourself by cutting your daily
  consumption in half. Substitute green tea or one of the SUPER BENEFICIAL
  herbal teas, such as hops, ginger, or sarsaparilla.

Exercise Regimen

- Plan to exercise at least 4 days this week, for 45 minutes each day.

  2 days: aerobic activity

  2 days: weights

- If you have joint impairment, start slowly and gradually increase your
  duration and intensity of activity. The important factor is consistency. Just
  do it—as much as you're able.

- Use your journal to detail the time, activity, distance, and amount of weight.
  Note the number of repetitions for each exercise.

> ▪ **WEEK 1 SUCCESS STRATEGY** ▪
> ## Digestive Health = Joint Health
>
> ▪ To reduce gastric inflammation, take 1 teaspoon of fresh ginger juice (available in health-food stores) several times a day.

Week 2

Blood Type Diet and Supplements

▪ Begin to eliminate the next level of AVOID foods—corn, potatoes, beans, and legumes.

▪ Eat at least 2 BENEFICIAL animal proteins every day, choosing from the meat, poultry, and seafood lists.

▪ Initially, it is best to avoid foods listed as NEUTRAL: Allowed Infrequently.

▪ Continue to incorporate SUPER BENEFICIAL foods into your daily diet.

▪ If you're a coffee drinker, continue to cut your coffee intake, replacing it with BENEFICIAL herbal teas. Drink a cup of green tea every morning.

▪ Manage your mealtimes to aid proper digestion. Avoid eating on the run. Make your meals relaxing, sit-down affairs. Eat slowly and chew thoroughly to encourage digestive secretions.

Exercise Regimen

▪ Continue to exercise at least 4 days this week for 45 minutes each day.

  2 days: aerobic activity

  2 days: weights

▪ If your work is sedentary, get in the habit of taking a couple of "movement" breaks during the day. Walk around the block or up and down stairs. Movement will help maintain joint flexibility.

> ▪ **WEEK 2 SUCCESS STRATEGY** ▪
> ## Tips for Type O Seniors
>
> Mobility is a primary issue for seniors, and this is especially true for Blood Type Os, who thrive on physical activity. Pay careful attention to the following strategies:
>
> ▪ Maintain a high-protein diet, using protein shakes as supplements, if you need to. Protein is the key for preventing arth-

ritis and inflammatory conditions, which are problems for Blood Type O. It is also the key for maintaining healthy bones and muscle mass.

- If you have painful rheumatoid arthritis or inflammation, avoid using non-steroidal anti-inflammatory drugs, such as ibuprofen and naprosin. These are known to cause peptic ulcers in Blood Type O patients.

- Think twice about undergoing elective surgery that might keep you off your feet for a few days. Studies show that for the average elderly person, one week of hospitalization is equivalent to one year of lost activity.

Week 3

Blood Type Diet and Supplements

- When you plan your meals for week 3, choose BENEFICIAL or SUPER BENEFICIAL foods to replace NEUTRAL foods whenever possible. For example, choose lean, organic beef or buffalo over chicken, or blueberries over an apple.

- Eliminate all remaining AVOID foods.

- Liberally incorporate SUPER BENEFICIAL foods into your daily diet.

- Completely wean yourself from coffee, substituting green or herbal tea.

Exercise Regimen

- Continue to exercise at least 4 days this week for 45 minutes each day.

  2 days: aerobic activity

  2 days: weights

▪WEEK 3 SUCCESS STRATEGY▪
Soothe Your Joints Naturally

Take a bath, as hot as you can tolerate, with Epsom salt (magnesium sulfate). Magnesium has anti-inflammatory and anti-arthritic properties, and it can be absorbed through the skin.

Week 4

Blood Type Diet and Supplements

- Continue at the week 3 level, focusing on BENEFICIAL and SUPER BENEFICIAL foods.
- Evaluate the first 4 weeks and make adjustments.

Exercise Regimen

- Continue at the week 3 level.
- Review your progress, noting in your journal improvements in strength and flexibility. Determine which exercise regimen has worked for you, including time of day, setting, and activity level.

■WEEK 4 SUCCESS STRATEGY■
Super-Acting Arthritis Herb

Stinging nettle leaf and root (*Urtica dioica*) appears to prevent overstimulation of pro-inflammatory molecules called cytokines. Cytokine balance is a growing topic of interest in medicine. In fact, virtually all immune disorders—HIV, cancer, allergies, autoimmune diseases, and even obesity/insulin resistance have characteristic imbalances in cytokine levels. Stinging nettle has a lectin with many unique characteristics. *Urtica dioica* agglutinin (UDA) has been shown to prevent the development of lupus in laboratory animals. Drinking 2 cups of stinging nettle leaf tea (available at health-food stores) every day can help reduce arthritis pain and inflammation.

A Final Word

In summary, the secret to fighting arthritis with the Blood Type O Diet involves:

1. Increasing fitness and active tissue mass by adhering to a diet that is animal protein–based.
2. Minimizing the consumption of pro-inflammatory lectins, most abundant in grains, such as wheat.

3. Increasing strength, flexibility, and circulatory efficiency by adopting a vigorous exercise program.
4. Using supplements to block the effects of pro-inflammatory lectins, provide antioxidant support, and help repair damaged tissue.

FIVE

Blood Type

A

BLOOD TYPE A DIET OUTCOME: SYSTEMIC RELIEF

"I have Still's disease, the systemic form of Juvenile Rheumatoid Arthritis. My first fever occurred three years ago today. I started the Type A Diet, and almost immediately felt a change in the nature of my constant fatigue."*

BLOOD TYPE DIET OUTCOME: PAIN-FREE, MED-FREE

"Last year I was forced to stop taking my NSAIDs for rheumatoid arthritis and go on a cleansing for a colon scan. Since I was off my medications I decided to try the Type A diet. I first stopped all nightshades and red meat. The change was dramatic. I continued to follow the diet closely and have not returned to medication since then. I am somewhat skeptical about this outcome since it is so significant. Perhaps I am experiencing a remission, and perhaps it is the diet. Whatever it is, I am without pain for the first time in ten years."

* Self-reported outcomes from the Blood Type Diet web site, www.dadamo.com

BLOOD TYPE A'S PATH TO ARTHRITIS INVOLVES THE OVER-stimulation of adhesion molecules (selectins) on the blood vessel walls, which allows excessive white blood cell migration into the tissues and triggers inflammation.

A diet low in animal protein and fats—especially red meat—is crucial strategy in Blood Type A's arthritis-fighting regimen, as high fat and protein diets increase levels of E-selectin which promotes inflammation, while soy and other vegetable proteins lower them.

Heart Attack Alert

NEW INFORMATION about about the connection between arthritis and an increased risk of heart attack has special importance for Blood Type A women. Researchers at the Brigham and Women's Hospital found that women with rheumatoid arthritis had twice the risk of heart attack compared to those without it. Those who had the joint condition for at least ten years faced triple the heart attack risks of nonsufferers. There is plenty of evidence that Blood Type A individuals who are overweight, have high cholesterol, and are diabetic place themselves at grave risk for heart attack. Now we see that there is an arthritis connection as well, and that connection is inflammation. All the more reason to eat the right diet for your type.

The Stress Factor

UNDER STRESSFUL SITUATIONS, Blood Type A manufactures higher levels of the stress hormone cortisol and has trouble clearing it from the body once the stressful event has passed. That means Blood Type A tends to be in a physiological state of stress, even when external circumstances are not stressful. High stress levels are implicated in many diseases, and research shows that it plays a role in the development of arthritis, as well as the severity of the condition.

One of the effects of high cortisol is a disruption of the sleep cy-

Blood Type A Arthritis-Fighting Food Analysis

ANTI-INFLAMMATORY FOODS	PRO-INFLAMMATORY FOODS
Soy foods	Red meat
Richly oiled cold water fish	Cow's milk–based dairy foods
Flax (linseed) oil	Corn, cottonseed, peanut oil
Olive oil	Kidney, navy beans
Onion	Wheat
Broccoli	White potatoes
Spinach, kale, collards	Bell peppers
Avocado	Eggplant
Pineapple	Tomato and tomato products
Blueberries, cherries, elderberries	Oranges
Ginger	Food additives
Turmeric	Processed sugar
Green tea	

cle, which, in turn places extra stress on the body. Studies show that many people with arthritic conditions such as fibromyalgia experience a type of sleep disturbance called alpha delta sleep disorder. People with alpha delta sleep disorder experience a disruption in sleep patterns. They don't obtain enough deep sleep—the phase in which muscles are repaired.

Musculoskeletal pain is also worsened by poor sleep. Most people who don't sleep well have muscle aches, regardless of the cause of their sleep disturbance.

Stress reduction can be a significant strategy for Blood Type A arthritis sufferers.

Glucosamine-Chondroitin and Blood Type A

SINCE THE INTRODUCTION of the "arthritis cure," many of my patients have wanted to know if they should take glucosamine and chondroitin. I have found that Blood Type A can effectively use these supplements when they do so in conjunction with the Blood Type Diet. Glucosamine helps to block inflammation-producing lectins, especially wheat germ lectin, by acting as a decoy. The lectin binds to it instead of binding to your intestinal lining.

While chondroitin is not recommended for every blood type, it provides special advantages for Blood Type A. Here's why. If we were to analyze the structure of chondroitin, we would see that it is composed of the repeating sugar N-acetyl galactosamine. N-acetyl galactosamine is the Blood Type A antigen. Thus, by consuming chondroitin as Blood Type A, you are adding a supportive element to your fight against arthritis.

Blood Type A individuals with rheumatoid arthritis may want to consider supplenting with a gamma linolenic acid (GLA) supplement. The best source of GLA is borage oil, which contain up to 24 percent GLA. Evening primrose oil (8–10 percent GLA) and black currant oil (15–17 percent GLA) are other good sources. I have found that Blood Type A seems to do best on the black currant seed oil source, usually six grams per day. The first positive effects of GLA on rheumatoid arthritis can generally be seen after one month of supplementation, with improvement continuing for a year or longer, suggesting that GLA may fuction as a slow-acting, disease-modifying antirheumatic drug. Studies have shown that borage oil is safe and non-toxic, even in large amounts.

Blood Type A: The Foods

THE BLOOD TYPE A Arthritis Diet is specifically adapted for the prevention and management of arthritis. A new category, **Super Beneficial**, highlights powerful arthritis-fighting foods for Blood Type A. The **Neutral** category has also been adjusted to de-emphasize foods that are less advantageous for you. Foods designated **Neutral: Allowed Infrequently** should be minimized or avoided entirely.

Your secretor status can influence your ability to fully digest and metabolize certain foods, so various adjustments in the values are made for non-secretors. If you do not know your secretor type, the odds are that you can safely use the "secretor" values, since the majority of the population (approximately 80 percent) are secretors. However, I urge you to get tested, since the variations are important for non-secretors who want to maximize the effectiveness of the Blood Type Diet.

The food charts are divided into three sections. The top of the chart suggests the average portion size and quantity per week or day, according to secretor status. These recommendations do *not* apply to the category **Neutral: Allowed Infrequently;** those foods should be eaten rarely, if at all. The charts also indicate differences in frequency

SUPER BENEFICIAL	Foods that are known to have specific disease-fighting qualities for your blood type.
BENEFICIAL	Foods with components that enhance the metabolic, immune, or structural health of you blood type.
NEUTRAL: Allowed Infrequently	Foods that normally have no direct type effect but may impede your progress when consumed regularly.
AVOID	Foods with components that are harmful to your blood type.

for some foods, based on ethnic heritage. It has been my experience that this factor has an impact upon the individual's ability to fully digest certain foods. For the purposes of blood type food choices, persons of Hispanic heritage should follow the recommendations for Caucasians, and North American Native peoples should follow the recommendations for Asians.

The middle section of the chart gives the food values. The bottom section lists variants based on secretor status.

For your convenience, we have included a number of product names (Ezekiel bread, Worcestershire sauce, etc.). However, keep in mind that commercial formulations vary among brands and regions. Even though a product may be listed as acceptable for you, always check its ingredients; do not use products that contain **Avoid** ingredients for your blood type. Of course, you may choose to make your own version of commercial products, such as bread and mayonnaise, using ingredients that suit your blood type. There are hundreds of delicious recipes for every blood type available on our Web site (www.dadamo. com) and in the book *Cook Right 4 Your Type: The Practical Kitchen Companion to* Eat Right 4 Your Type.

Meat/Poultry

Many of the diseases related to a high-fat diet are more common in Blood Type A than in the other blood types. Blood Type A lacks some of the enzymes and stomach acids needed to effectively digest animal protein. When you overconsume meat, the undigested by-products can create a toxic environment. Many inflammatory conditions are the result of the ensuing gastrointestinal conditions. For this reason you should derive most of your protein from non-meat sources. Non-secretors have a small advantage over secretors in the ability to digest animal protein but should still derive most of their protein from foods other than meat. Choose only the best-quality (preferably free-range), chemical-, antibiotic-, and pesticide-free, low-fat meats and poultry.

BLOOD TYPE A: MEAT/POULTRY			
Portion: 4–6 oz (men); 2–5 oz (women and children)			
	African	**Caucasian**	**Asian**
Secretor	0–2	0–3	0–3
Non-Secretor	2–5	2–4	2–3
		Times per week	

SUPER BENEFICIAL	BENEFICIAL	NEUTRAL: Allowed Frequently	NEUTRAL: Allowed Infrequently	AVOID
		Chicken Cornish hen Grouse Guinea hen Ostrich Squab Turkey		All commercially processed meats Bacon/Ham/Pork Beef Buffalo Duck Goat Goose Heart (beef) Horse Lamb Liver (calf) Mutton Partridge Pheasant Quail Rabbit Squirrel Sweetbreads Turtle Veal Venison

Special Variants: *Non-Secretor* BENEFICIAL: turkey; NEUTRAL (Allowed Frequently): duck, goat, goose, lamb, mutton, partridge, pheasant, quail, rabbit, turtle.

Fish/Seafood

Fish and seafood represent a nutritious source of protein for Blood Type A. SUPER BENEFICIAL are the richly oiled cold-water fish, such as cod, mackerel, salmon, trout, and sardines. These are rich in omega-3 fatty acids, such as docosahexaenoic acid (DHA) and eicosapentaenoic acid (EPA), which can help to balance immune function and reduce inflammation.

BLOOD TYPE A: FISH/SEAFOOD			
Portion: 4–6 oz (men); 2–5 oz (women and children)			
	African	Caucasian	Asian
Secretor	1–3	1–3	1–3
Non-Secretor	2–5	2–5	2–4
		Times per week	

SUPER BENEFICIAL	BENEFICIAL	NEUTRAL: Allowed Frequently	NEUTRAL: Allowed Infrequently	AVOID
Cod	Carp	Abalone		Anchovy
Mackerel	Monkfish	Bass (sea)		Barracuda
Salmon	Perch	Bullhead		Bass
Sardine	(silver/	Butterfish		(bluegill/
Trout (rain-	yellow)	Chub		striped)
bow/ sea)	Pickerel	Croaker		Beluga
	Pollock	Cusk		Bluefish
	Red	Drum		Catfish
	Snapper	Halfmoon		Caviar
	Snail (*Helix*	fish		(sturgeon)
	Pomatia/	Mahi-mahi		Clam
	escargot)	Mullet		Conch
	Whitefish	Muskel-		Crab
	Whiting	lunge		Eel
		Orange		Flounder
		roughy		Frog
		Parrot fish		Gray sole

SUPER BENEFICIAL	BENEFICIAL	NEUTRAL: Allowed Frequently	NEUTRAL: Allowed Infrequently	AVOID
		Perch (ocean/ white)		Grouper
		Pike		Haddock
		Pompano		Hake
		Porgy		Halibut
		Rosefish		Harvest fish
		Sailfish		Herring
		Salmon roe		(fresh/
		Scrod		pickled/
		Shark		smoked)
		Smelt		Lobster
		Snapper		Mussels
		Sturgeon		Octopus
		Sucker		Opaleye fish
		Sunfish		Oyster
		Swordfish		Salmon
		Tilapia		(smoked)
		Trout		Scallops
		(brook)		Scup
		Tuna		Shad
		Weakfish		Shrimp
		Yellowtail		Sole
				Squid
				(calamari)
				Tilefish

Special Variants: *Non-Secretor* BENEFICIAL: chub, cusk, drum, halfmoon fish, harvest fish, mullet, muskellunge, perch (white), pompano, rosefish, sailfish, sucker, swordfish, trout (brook); NEUTRAL (Allowed Frequently): anchovy, bass (bluegill), beluga, bluefish, caviar (sturgeon), flounder, frog, gray sole, grouper, haddock, hake, halibut, herring (fresh), mussels, octopus, opaleye fish, scallops, scup, shad, tilefish.

Dairy/Eggs

Blood Type A may consume small quantities of dairy foods but should limit your intake of cow's milk–derived products. Be especially cautious if you suffer from allergies or other inflammatory conditions; these can be exacerbated by dairy. Eggs can be consumed in moderation. They are a good source of docosahexaenoic acid (DHA). However, for most Blood Type A individuals, fish is the preferred source of DHA over eggs, since Blood Type A is associated with greater sensitivity to dietary sources of cholesterol than the other blood types. Do your best to find eggs and dairy products that meet organic standards.

BLOOD TYPE A: EGGS			
Portion: 1 egg			
	African	**Caucasian**	**Asian**
Secretor	1–3	1–3	1–3
Non-Secretor	2–3	2–5	2–4
		Times per week	

BLOOD TYPE A: MILK AND YOGURT			
Portion: 4–6 oz (men); 2–5 oz (women and children)			
	African	**Caucasian**	**Asian**
Secretor	0–1	1–3	0–3
Non-Secretor	0–1	1–2	0–2
		Times per week	

BLOOD TYPE A: CHEESE			
Portion: 3 oz (men); 2 oz (women and children)			
	African	**Caucasian**	**Asian**
Secretor	0–2	1–3	0–2
Non-Secretor	0	0–1	0–1
		Times per week	

SUPER BENEFICIAL	BENEFICIAL	NEUTRAL: Allowed Frequently	NEUTRAL: Allowed Infrequently	AVOID
		Egg (chicken/ duck/ goose/ quail) Farmer cheese Feta Ghee (clarified butter) Goat cheese Kefir Milk (goat) Mozzarella Paneer Ricotta Sour cream Yogurt		American cheese Blue cheese Brie Butter Buttermilk Camembert Casein Cheddar Colby Cottage cheese Cream cheese Edam Emmenthal Gouda Gruyère Half-and-half Ice cream Jarlsberg Milk (cow) Monterey Jack Muenster Neufchâtel Parmesan Provolone Quark Sherbet Swiss cheese Whey

Special Variants: *Non-Secretor* NEUTRAL (Allowed Frequently): cottage cheese, whey; AVOID: milk (goat), sour cream.

Oils

Olive oil, a monounsaturated fat, is SUPER BENEFICIAL for Blood Type A. Constituents in olive oil, such as flavonoids, squalenes, and polyphenols, act as powerful antioxidants. Use it as your primary cooking oil. Also SUPER BENEFICIAL is flax oil (linseed), which is high in alpha-linolenic acid (ALA) and has anti-inflammatory properties.

Some research suggests that the components of avocado and soybean oils might cause positive changes in the cartilage-producing cells (chondrocytes) of people with osteoarthritis. In a study published in the *Journal of Rheumatology*, the oils, either in combination or individually, enhanced the production of chondrocytes of aggrecan, a key component of cartilage, beginning after nine days of treatment and increasing through day twelve.

Be aware that some oils are high in omega-6 fatty acids, which can stimulate the inflammatory response. These include corn, cottonseed, and peanut oils.

BLOOD TYPE A: OILS			
Portion: 1 tblsp			
	African	Caucasian	Asian
Secretor	5–8	5–8	5–8
Non-Secretor	3–7	3–7	3–6
	Times per week		

SUPER BENEFICIAL	BENEFICIAL	NEUTRAL: Allowed Frequently	NEUTRAL: Allowed Infrequently	AVOID
Flax (linseed) Olive	Black currant seed Soy bean Walnut	Almond Avocado Borage seed Canola Cod liver Evening primrose Sesame	Safflower Sunflower Wheat germ	Castor Coconut Corn Cottonseed Peanut

Special Variants: *Non-Secretor* BENEFICIAL: cod liver, sesame; NEUTRAL (Allowed Frequently): peanut; AVOID: safflower.

Nuts and Seeds

Nuts and seeds can serve as an important secondary source of protein for Blood Type A. Laboratory research has identified at least five natural phytochemicals in nuts that regulate the immune system and act as antioxidants. SUPER BENEFICIAL for Blood Type A are flaxseeds and walnuts, which are high in omega-3 fatty acids. Flaxseeds are particularly rich in lignans, which can help lower the number of receptors for epidermal growth factor. High levels of EGF can trigger inflammatory conditions.

BLOOD TYPE A: NUTS AND SEEDS			
Portion: Whole (handful); Nut Butters (2 tblsp)			
	African	**Caucasian**	**Asian**
Secretor	4–7	4–7	4–7
Non-Secretor	5–7	5–7	5–7
		Times per week	

SUPER BENEFICIAL	BENEFICIAL	NEUTRAL: Allowed Frequently	NEUTRAL: Allowed Infrequently	AVOID
Flax (linseed) Walnut (black/ English)	Peanut Peanut butter Pumpkin seed	Almond Almond butter Almond cheese Almond milk Beechnut Butternut Chestnut Filbert (hazelnut) Hickory nut Litchi	Safflower seed Sesame butter (tahini) Sesame seed Sunflower butter Sunflower seed	Brazil nut Cashew Pistachio

SUPER BENEFICIAL	BENEFICIAL	NEUTRAL: Allowed Frequently	NEUTRAL: Allowed Infrequently	AVOID
		Macadamia nut Pecan Pignolia (pine nut) Poppy seed		

Special Variants: *Non-Secretor* AVOID: safflower seed, sunflower butter, sunflower seed.

Beans and Legumes

Blood Type A thrives on vegetable proteins found in many beans and legumes, although a few beans contain immunoreactive proteins and should be avoided. SUPER BENEFICIAL beans and legumes for Blood Type A include soy beans and their by-products. They are a good source of essential amino acids, and they contain isoflavones that can inhibit inflammation-producing selectins from being over-expressed in the blood vessels.

BLOOD TYPE A: BEANS AND LEGUMES			
Portion: 1 cup (cooked)			
	African	Caucasian	Asian
Secretor	5–7	5–7	5–7
Non-Secretor	3–5	3–5	3–5
		Times per week	

SUPER BENEFICIAL	BENEFICIAL	NEUTRAL: Allowed Frequently	NEUTRAL: Allowed Infrequently	AVOID
Miso Soy bean Soy cheese Soy milk Tempeh Tofu	Adzuki bean Bean (green/snap/string) Black bean Black-eyed pea Fava (broad) bean Lentil (all) Pinto bean	Cannellini bean Jicama bean Lima bean Mung bean/sprouts Northern bean Pea (green/pod/snow) White bean		Copper bean Garbanzo (chickpea) Kidney bean Navy bean Tamarind bean

Special Variants: *Non-Secretor* NEUTRAL (Allowed Frequently): adzuki bean, bean (green/snap/string), black bean, black-eyed pea, copper bean, fava (broad) bean, kidney bean, navy bean.

Grains and Starches

Blood Type A benefits from a moderate consumption of grains. If you have arthritis, you should limit or avoid wheat and corn products. This is especially important for non-secretors. The agglutinin in whole wheat can aggravate inflammatory conditions and derail the proper response of the immune system. This lectin can sometimes be milled out of the grain or destroyed by sprouting.

BLOOD TYPE A: GRAINS AND STARCHES			
Portion: ½ cup dry (grains or pastas); 1 muffin; 2 slices of bread			
	African	Caucasian	Asian
Secretor	7–10	7–9	7–10
Non-Secretor	5–7	5–7	5–7
		Times per week	

SUPER BENEFICIAL	BENEFICIAL	NEUTRAL: Allowed Frequently	NEUTRAL: Allowed Infrequently	AVOID
	Amaranth	Barley	Cornmeal	Teff
	Buckwheat	Grits	Couscous	Wheat bran
	Essene	Kamut	Millet	Wheat germ
	bread	Quinoa	Popcorn	
	(manna)	Rice (wild)	Tapioca	
	Ezekiel	Sorghum	Wheat	
	bread	Spelt	(whole)	
	Oat bran	(whole)		
	Oat flour	Spelt		
	Oatmeal	flour/		
	Rice	products		
	Rice bran	Wheat (re-		
	Rice cake	fined/un-		
	Rice flour	bleached)		
	Rice milk	Wheat (se-		
	Rye (whole)	molina)		
	Rye flour/	Wheat		
	products	(white		
	Soba	flour)		
	noodles	100%		
	(100%	sprouted		
	buck-	grain		
	wheat)	products		
	Soy flour/	(except		
	products	Essene,		
		Ezekiel)		

Special Variants: *Non-Secretor* NEUTRAL (Allowed Frequently): buckwheat, rice cake, soba noodles (100% buckwheat), soy flour/products, teff; AVOID: cornmeal, couscous, popcorn, wheat (all).

Vegetables

Vegetables can be your first line of defense against chronic disease. They provide a rich source of antioxidants and fiber and are essential to intestinal health. Many are high in potassium, which is especially critical if you are taking NSAIDs. Blood Type A SUPER BENEFI-CIALS include onions and garlic, which are high in quercetin, a flavonoid with potent anti-inflammatory properties, and other antioxidants that decrease oxidative stress and increase glutathione, which protects cells. Onions and garlic are also rich sources of diallyl sulfide, which detoxifies carcinogens. Broccoli contains allyl methyl trisulfide and dithiolthiones, which increase the activity of enzymes involved in detoxification of carcinogens. Spinach, kale, and Swiss chard contain potent antioxidants. Celery can help reduce the inflammation of arthritis.

Tomatoes contain a lectin that reacts negatively with the saliva and digestive juices of Blood Type A secretors, although it does not appear to react with non-secretors. Yams are typically high in the amino acid phenylalanine, which inactivates intestinal alkaline phosphatase (already quite low in Blood Type A) and should be minimized or avoided completely. Corn should be minimized or avoided if you have arthritis.

An item's value also applies to its juice, unless otherwise noted.

BLOOD TYPE A: VEGETABLES			
Portion: 1 cup, prepared (cooked or raw)			
	African	**Caucasian**	**Asian**
Secretor Super/ Beneficials	Unlimited	Unlimited	Unlimited
Secretor Neutrals	2–5	2–5	2–5
Non-Secretor Super/ Beneficials	Unlimited	Unlimited	Unlimited
Non-Secretor Neutrals	2–3	2–3	2–3
	Times per day		

SUPER BENEFICIAL	BENEFICIAL	NEUTRAL: Allowed Frequently	NEUTRAL: Allowed Infrequently	AVOID
Broccoli Celery Garlic Kale Onion (all) Spinach Swiss chard	Alfalfa sprouts Aloe Artichoke Beet greens Carrot Cauliflower Chicory Collards Dandelion Escarole Horseradish Kohlrabi Leek Lettuce (Romaine) Mushroom (maitake/silver dollar) Okra Parsnip Pumpkin Rappini (broccoli rabe) Turnip	Arugula Asparagus Asparagus pea Bamboo shoot Beet Bok choy Brussels sprouts Cabbage (juice)* Cauliflower Celeriac Cucumber Daikon radish Endive Fennel Fiddlehead fern Lettuce (except Romaine) Mushroom (abalone/enoki/oyster/portobello/straw/tree ear) Mustard greens Oyster plant	Corn Olive (green) Pickles (in brine) Squash (all)	Cabbage Eggplant Mushroom (shiitake) Olive (black/Greek/Spanish) Peppers (all) Pickles (in vinegar) Potato Potato (sweet) Rhubarb Tomato Yam Yucca

SUPER BENEFICIAL	BENEFICIAL	NEUTRAL: Allowed Frequently	NEUTRAL: Allowed Infrequently	AVOID

		Poi
		Radicchio
		Radish/
		  sprouts
		Rutabaga
		Scallion
		Seaweeds
		Shallot
		Squash
		  (all)
		Taro
		Water
		  chestnut
		Watercress
		Zucchini		

Special Variants: *Non-Secretor* NEUTRAL (Allowed Frequently): alfalfa sprouts, aloe, carrot, fennel, garlic, horseradish, lettuce (Romaine), mushroom (maitake/ shiitake), potato (sweet), rappini (broccoli rabe), taro, tomato; AVOID: agar, cabbage (juice),*mushroom (silver dollar), olive (green), pickles (in brine).

*To obtain the benefits of cabbage juice, it must be consumed within one minute of juicing.

Fruits and Fruit Juices

Fruits are rich in antioxidants and many, such as blueberries, elderberries, cherries, and blackberries, are high in anthocyanins, which enhance collagen integrity. Pineapple contains bromelain, a powerful enzyme that has an anti-inflammatory effect on muscle and tissue. Pineapple is also a good source of vitamin C, a deficiency of which is seen in many cases of arthritis. Red grapefruit and watermelon supply the antioxidant lycopene, in lieu of using tomatoes. Plums and prunes are high in the phytonutrients neochlorogenic and chlorogenic acid. These substances are classified as phenols, and their function as antioxidants has been well documented. Several fruits, such as bananas and oranges, contain Blood Type A reactive lectins and should be avoided.

An item's value also applies to its juice, unless otherwise noted.

BLOOD TYPE A: FRUITS AND FRUIT JUICES			
Portion: 1 cup			
	African	Caucasian	Asian
Secretor	2–4	3–4	3–4
Non-Secretor	2–3	2–3	2–3
		Times per day	

SUPER BENEFICIAL	BENEFICIAL	NEUTRAL: Allowed Frequently	NEUTRAL: Allowed Infrequently	AVOID
Blueberry	Apricot	Apple	Currant	Banana
Cherry (all)	Blackberry	Asian pear	Date	Bitter melon
Elderberry	Boysen-	Avocado	Quince	Coconut
(dark	berry	Breadfruit	Raisin	Honeydew
blue/	Cranberry	Canang	Star fruit	melon
purple)	Fig (fresh/	melon	(caram-	Mango
Grapefruit	dried)	Cantaloupe	bola)	Orange
(red)	Grapefruit	Casaba	Strawberry	Papaya
Pineapple	(white)	melon		Plantain
Plum (all)	Lemon	Christmas		Tangerine
Prune	Lime	melon		
Water-		Cranberry		
melon		(juice)		
		Crenshaw		
		melon		
		Dewberry		
		Goose-		
		berry		
		Grape (all)		
		Guava		
		Kiwi		
		Kumquat		
		Logan-		
		berry		

SUPER BENEFICIAL	BENEFICIAL	NEUTRAL: Allowed Frequently	NEUTRAL: Allowed Infrequently	AVOID

		Mulberry
		Musk-
		  melon
		Nectarine
		Peach
		Pear
		Persian
		  melon
		Persimmon
		Pome-
		  granate
		Prickly
		  pear
		Raspberry
		Sago palm
		Spanish
		  melon
		Young-
		  berry		

Special Variants: Non-Secretor BENEFICIAL: cranberry (juice); NEUTRAL (Allowed Frequently): banana, lime, mango, plantain; AVOID: cantaloupe, casaba melon.

Spices/Condiments/Sweeteners

Many spices are known to have anti-inflammatory properties. The common cooking spices—rosemary, thyme, and oregano—are powerful antioxidants that exert anti-inflammatory effects. Turmeric and garlic are also anti-inflammatory. Ginger inhibits the production of COX-2, an enzyme that triggers the inflammatory response. Parsley contains quercetin, which is anti-inflammatory. Baker's and brewer's yeast are BENEFICIAL foods for Blood Type A non-secretors, enhancing glucose metabolism and helping to ensure a healthy flora balance in the intestinal tract. However, it should be minimized if you suffer from gout.

Many common food additives, such as guar gum and carrageenan, enhance the effects of lectins found in other foods and should be avoided. Use caution when using prepared condiments. They often contain wheat, which is a primary factor in the development of arthritis and other inflammatory conditions.

SUPER BENEFICIAL	BENEFICIAL	NEUTRAL: Allowed Frequently	NEUTRAL: Allowed Infrequently	AVOID
Dill	Apple	Agar	Brown rice	Aspartame
Garlic	pectin	Allspice	syrup	Capers
Ginger	Barley malt	Almond	Chocolate	Carrageenan
Oregano	Fenugreek	extract	Cornstarch	Chili powder
Rosemary	Horse-	Anise	Corn syrup	Gelatin (ex-
Thyme	radish	Arrowroot	Dextrose	cept veg-
Turmeric	Molasses	Basil	Fructose	sourced)
	(black-	Bay leaf	Guarana	Gums (aca-
	strap)	Bergamot	Honey	cia/Arabic/
	Mustard	Caraway	Malto-	guar)
	(dry)	Cardamon	dextrin	Juniper
	Parsley	Carob	Maple	Ketchup
	Soy sauce	Chervil	syrup	Mayonnaise
	(wheat-	Chive	Rice syrup	MSG
	free)	Cilantro	Senna	Pepper
	Tamari	(coriander	Sugar	(black/
	(wheat-	leaf)	(brown/	white)
	free)	Cinnamon	white)	Pepper
	Tarragon	Clove		(cayenne)
		Coriander		Pepper (pep-
		Cream of		percorn/
		tartar		red flakes)
		Cumin		Pickles/
		Invert		relish
		sugar		Sucanat
		Lecithin		Vinegar (all)
		Licorice		Wintergreen
		root*		
		Mace		

SUPER BENEFICIAL	BENEFICIAL	NEUTRAL: Allowed Frequently	NEUTRAL: Allowed Infrequently	AVOID
		Marjoram		
		Mint (all)		
		Molasses		
		Nutmeg		
		Paprika		
		Saffron		
		Sage		
		Savory		
		Sea salt		
		Seaweeds		
		Stevia		
		Tamarind		
		Vanilla		
		Vegetable glycerine		
		Yeast (baker's/ brewer's)		

Special Variants: *Non-Secretor* BENEFICIAL: cilantro (coriander leaf), yeast (brewer's); NEUTRAL (Allowed Frequently): barley malt, chili powder, dill, molasses, parsley, rice syrup, soy sauce (wheat-free), tamari (wheat-free), wintergreen; AVOID: agar, cornstarch, corn syrup, dextrose, invert sugar, maltodextrin, senna.

* Do not use if you have high blood pressure.

Herbal Teas

Several herbal teas can be SUPER BENEFICIAL arthritis fighters for Blood Type A. Many herbal teas are anti-inflammatory. These include ginger, fenugreek, and holy basil. Echinacea and rosehip can support immune health.

SUPER BENEFICIAL	BENEFICIAL	NEUTRAL: Allowed Frequently	NEUTRAL: Allowed Infrequently	AVOID
Echinacea	Aloe	Chickweed	Hops	Catnip
Fenugreek	Alfalfa	Coltsfoot	Senna	Corn silk
Ginger	Burdock	Dong quai		Pepper
Holy basil	Chamomile	Elderberry		(cayenne)
Rosehip	Dandelion	Goldenseal		Red clover
	Gentian	Horehound		Rhubarb
	Ginkgo	Licorice		Yellow dock
	biloba	root*		
	Ginseng	Linden		
	Hawthorn	Mulberry		
	Milk thistle	Mullein		
	Parsley	Pepper-		
	Slippery	mint		
	elm	Raspberry		
	St. John's	leaf		
	wort	Sage		
	Stone root	Sarsaparilla		
	Valerian	Shepherd's		
		purse		
		Skullcap		
		Spearmint		
		Strawberry		
		leaf		
		Thyme		
		White birch		
		White oak		
		bark		
		Yarrow		

Special Variants: *Non-Secretor* AVOID: senna.

* Do not use if you have high blood pressure.

Miscellaneous Beverages

Green tea is a SUPER BENEFICIAL beverage for Blood Type A because of its antioxidant properties. Red wine contains gallic acid, transresveratrol, quercetin, and rutin—four phenolic compounds with potent antioxidant effects. Blood Type A individuals who are not caffeine sensitive might consider having one cup of coffee daily; it contains many enzymes also found in soy, which can help your immune system function more effectively.

SUPER BENEFICIAL	BENEFICIAL	NEUTRAL: Allowed Frequently	NEUTRAL: Allowed Infrequently	AVOID
Tea (green) Wine (red)	Coffee (regular)	Coffee (decaf) Wine (white)		Beer Liquor Seltzer Soda (club) Soda (cola/ diet/misc.) Tea, black (reg/decaf)

Special Variants: *Non-Secretor* BENEFICIAL: wine (white); NEUTRAL (Allowed Frequently): seltzer, tea (black: reg/decaf).

Supplements

THE BLOOD TYPE A DIET offers abundant quantities of important nutrients, such as protein and iron. It is important to get as many nutrients as possible from fresh foods and use supplements only to fill in the minor deficiencies in your diet. The following supplement protocols are designed for Blood Type A individuals who are suffering from arthritis or related autoimmune conditions.

Note: If you are being treated for a medical condition, consult your doctor before taking any supplements.

Blood Type A: Anti-Inflammatory Protocol

Use this protocol for 12 weeks to prevent and minimize inflammatory conditions, while balancing immune function.

SUPPLEMENT	ACTION	DOSAGE
Chondroitin sulfate	Supports regeneration of bone cartilage	600 mg, 2 capsules daily, away from food
Glucosamine sulfate	Enables joint repair	500 mg, 2–3 capsules daily, away from food
Frankincense (*Boswellia Serrata*)	Has anti-inflammatory effects	500 mg, 1–2 capsules between meals
Larch arabinogalactan (*Larix officinalis*)	Promotes digestive and intestinal health	1 tablespoon, twice daily, in juice or water
Quercetin	Has anti-inflammatory effects	500 mg, twice daily, away from food
GLA supplement (such as one made from black currant seed oil)	Balances anti- and pro-inflammatory in immune system	3–6 grams daily
Ginger root (*Rhizome zingiberis*)	*COX-2 inhibitor; arthritis pain reliever; digestive aid*	*200 mg capsule before food, as a tea or compress*

Blood Type A: Arthritis Pain Relief Adjunct

Use this protocol for 4 weeks to reduce pain associated with joint disease.

SUPPLEMENT	ACTION	DOSAGE
Ginger root (*Rhizome zingiberis*)	COX-2 inhibitor; pain reliever	200 mg capsule before meals, as a tea or compress
Bromelain (pineapple enzyme)	Has antioxidant and anti-inflammatory properties	500 mg, 1–3 capsules daily with meals, gradually decreasing dose and frequency as symptoms improve

Blood Type A: Joint Repair Adjunct

Use this protocol for 4 weeks to promote healing and improve joint integrity.

SUPPLEMENT	ACTION	DOSAGE
Chondroitin sulfate	Supports regeneration of joint cartilage	600 mg, 2 capsules daily, away from food
Glucosamine sulfate	Enables joint repair	500 mg, twice daily, away from food
Vitamin C (rose hips or acerola cherry)	Powerful antioxidant; promotes healing	250 mg, twice daily

Blood Type A: Surgery Recovery Adjunct

When surgery is scheduled, add this protocol for 2 weeks before surgery and 2 weeks after.

SUPPLEMENT	ACTION	DOSAGE
Gotu kola (*Centella asiatica*)*	Aids wound healing and proper blood flow	100 mg, twice daily
Vitamin E	Powerful antioxidant; aids wound healing	400 IU daily
Horse chestnut (*Aesculus hippocastanum*)	Has anti-inflammatory properties	500 mg, twice daily
Chamomile (*Matricaria chamomilla*)	A mild digestive and antidepressant	Herbal tincture: 25 drops in warm water, 2–3 times daily

*Do not use if you are pregnant.

The Exercise Component

FOR BLOOD TYPE A, stress regulation and overall fitness depend on engaging in regular exercises, with an emphasis on calming exercises such as Hatha yoga and T'ai Chi, as well as light aerobic exercise such as walking. These guidelines are perfectly suited to the needs of Blood Type A individuals suffering from arthritis.

Done properly, yoga can be especially effective for arthritis relief. This ancient system of exercise uses special postures to stretch, strengthen, and align the body. Yoga also uses breathing exercises and meditation to focus the mind and promote relaxation. If you have arthritis, a gentle yoga program may be a great way to keep moving without putting too much strain on your joints. Be sure to find an instructor who is trained to work with arthritic conditions. There are several different styles of yoga, so you need to choose the one that works for your condition.

T'ai Chi, a martial art that is basically a form of moving meditation, can gently improve range of motion for arthritis sufferers. T'ai Chi also helps to reduce stress, lower blood pressure, and improve mood.

Walking or brisk walking is the ideal aerobic exercise for Blood Type A, especially when you walk outdoors in a quiet, natural setting. Studies consistently show that light aerobic exercise can reduce joint swelling. Physical exercise also promotes lean muscle mass and reduces weight, thus lightening the load on stressed joints.

The following comprises the ideal exercise regimen for Blood Type A:

EXERCISE	DURATION	FREQUENCY
Hatha yoga	40–50 minutes	3–4 x week
T'ai Chi	40–50 minutes	3–4 x week
Aerobics (low-impact)	40–50 minutes	2–3 x week
Treadmill	30 minutes	2–3 x week
Pilates	40–50 minutes	3–4 x week
Weight training (5–10 lb free weights)	15 minutes	2–3 x week
Cycling (recumbent bike)	30 minutes	2–3 x week
Swimming	30 minutes	2–3 x week
Brisk walking	45 minutes	2–3 x week

Getting Started: The First Month

IF YOU ARE NEW to the Blood Type Diet, the following guidelines will introduce you to the Blood Type A regimen over a period of one month. Follow these recommendations as closely as possible, using a journal to record your personal experiences with the diet. In addition to factors that are measurable in laboratory tests, take the time to note changes in your energy levels, pain levels, sleep patterns, digestion, and overall well-being.

Blood Type A Arthritis Diet Checklist

Avoid meat. Low levels of hydrochloric acid and intestinal ☐
alkaline phosphatase make it indigestible for Blood Type A.

Derive your primary protein from soy foods. ☐

Include regular portions of richly oiled cold-water fish every ☐
week.

Include modest amounts of cultured dairy foods in your diet ☐
but avoid fresh milk products, which cause excess mucus
production and can trigger inflammation.

Eat your beans—beans provide an essential high-protein vege- ☐
table source for Blood Type A.

Don't overdo the grains, especially wheat-derived foods. ☐
Avoid wheat if you have arthritis.

Eat lots of BENEFICIAL fruits and vegetables, especially those ☐
high in antioxidants and fiber.

Drink green tea every day for extra immune system benefits. ☐

Week 1

Blood Type Diet and Supplements

- Eliminate your most harmful AVOID foods—red meat, most dairy, and negative lectin-containing nuts, beans, and seeds.

- Include your most important BENEFICIAL foods frequently throughout the
  week. For example, have soy-based foods 5 times and omega-3-rich fish
  3 to 4 times, with lots of BENEFICIAL vegetables and fruit.

- Incorporate at least 1 SUPER BENEFICIAL food into your daily diet. For
  example, have a bowl of cherries as a snack, or a spinach salad with walnuts.

- If you have arthritis, avoid whole-wheat products.

- Drink 2 to 3 cups of green tea every day.

Exercise Regimen

- Plan to exercise at least 4 days this week, for 45 minutes each day.

  2 days: walking or light aerobic activity

  2 days: yoga or T'ai Chi

- If you have joint impairment, start slowly and gradually increase your duration and intensity of activity. The important factor is consistency. Just do it—as much as you're able.

- Use your journal to detail the time, activity, distance, and amount of weight. Note the number of repetitions for each exercise.

▪ WEEK 3 SUCCESS STRATEGY ▪
Green Tea–Lime Slushie

Here's a super way to drink your green tea, especially during warm weather.

1 quart brewed green tea
Pinch each of cinnamon, ginger, and tarragon
¼ cup maple syrup
Juice of 2 limes + 1 tsp lime zest

Mix ingredients and freeze in ice cube trays. To drink, blend to slushie consistency.

Week 2

Blood Type Diet and Supplements

- Begin to eliminate the next level of AVOID foods—grains, vegetables, and fruits that react poorly with Type A blood.

- Eat 2 to 3 BENEFICIAL proteins every day, with special emphasis on soy. Eat omega-3-rich fish at least 3 times a week.

- Continue to incorporate SUPER BENEFICIAL foods into your daily diet.

- Choose the NEUTRAL foods listed as Allowed Frequently, over those listed as Allowed Infrequently.

- Manage your mealtimes to aid proper digestion. Avoid eating on the run. Make your meals relaxing, sit-down affairs. Eat slowly and chew thoroughly to encourage digestive secretions.

Exercise Regimen

- Continue to exercise at least 4 days this week, for 45 minutes each day.
  2 days: walking or light aerobic activity
  2 days: yoga or T'ai Chi

- If your work is sedentary, get in the habit of taking a couple of "movement" breaks during the day. Walk around the block or up and down stairs. Movement will help maintain joint flexibility.

Sleep Tight

If stress and discomfort from arthritis have disrupted your sleep patterns, two supplements might help.

Methylcobalamin (active vitamin B$_{12}$): 1 to 3 mg per day taken in the morning. This vitamin enables deep sleep and helps you wake feeling more rested.

Melatonin: Melatonin is a hormone and should be taken only under a health professional's direction. In my experience, it is usually safe for Blood Type A and can benefit you in other ways—e.g., by alleviating EGF receptor overexpression and by improving immune function. However, using hormones as supplements should only be considered when other, gentler measures have failed.

Week 3

Blood Type Diet and Supplements

- When you plan your meals for week 3, choose BENEFICIAL foods to replace NEUTRAL foods whenever possible. For example, choose tofu over chicken, or blueberries over an apple.
- Eliminate all remaining AVOID foods.
- Liberally incorporate SUPER BENEFICIAL foods into your daily diet.
- Drink 2 to 3 cups of green tea every day.

Exercise Regimen

- Continue to exercise at least 4 days this week, for 45 minutes each day.
  2 days: walking or light aerobic activity
  2 days: yoga or T'ai Chi

Modify the Expression of Epidermal Growth Factor

Epidermal growth factor (EGF) has a tendency to be overexpressed in Blood Type A, creating inflammatory conditions. Here are some tips for modifying its expression:

- Reduce the amount of fat in your diet, especially the essential polyunsaturated fatty acid linoleic acid.

- Take a melatonin supplement before bedtime. Melatonin inhibits the uptake of plasma linoleic acid.
- Inhibit the activity of 5-lipoxygenase, a compound that promotes cellular growth. Olive oil is a 5-lipoxygenase inhibitor, as are active compounds in ginger, turmeric, stinging nettle, and rosemary.
- The antioxidants quercetin and luteolin appear to inhibit the stimulatory effects of EGF, probably by inhibiting its activity on the EGF receptor.

Week 4

Blood Type Diet and Supplements

- Continue at the week 3 level, focusing on BENEFICIAL and SUPER BENEFICIAL foods.

Exercise Regimen

- Continue at the week 3 level.

- Review your progress, noting in your journal improvements in strength and flexibility. Determine which exercise regimen has worked for you, including time of day, setting, and activity level.

■ WEEK 4 SUCCESS STRATEGY ■
Build Strong Bones

Type A women have an increased risk of bone loss as they age because of low levels of intestinal alkaline phosphatase. Repeated studies have shown that this enzyme positively impacts calcium metabolism. Furthermore, higher stomach acid predicts better calcium absorption. Although conventional wisdom in the nutrition community holds that high-protein diets accelerate bone loss, the scientific literature shows that the opposite is true. This presents a special challenge for Type A women. To promote healthy bones:

1. Eat canned salmon and sardines with the bones.
2. Regularly consume low-fat yogurt, soy milk, and goat milk.

3. Include lots of broccoli and spinach in your diet.
4. Take a daily dose of supplemental calcium citrate—300 to 600 mg.
5. Follow the Type A exercise regimen and do as much walking as you can.

A Final Word

IN SUMMARY, the secret to fighting arthritis with the Blood Type A Diet involves:

1. Increasing overall health and fitness by eating a diet rich in soy protein, BENEFICIAL seafood, and green vegetables.
2. Minimizing the consumption of pro-inflammatory lectins abundant in certain grains, beans, and vegetables that are not right for your type.
3. Regulating the effects of inflammatory molecules by avoiding red meat and high-fat foods.
4. Building strength and reducing stress by engaging in regular exercise appropriate for your blood type.
5. Using supplements to block the effects of pro-inflammatory lectins, provide antioxidant support, and help repair damaged tissue.

Blood Type

B

BLOOD TYPE OUTCOME: THE PAIN IS GONE

"I had arthritis in my left hip that hurt constantly and even made it hard
for me to get out of bed. The pain made me wince many times each day,
just doing the usual things. The Type B Diet has changed that. About
two weeks ago, I noticed that the pain was less. Within a few days, it was
all but gone. I'm talking about pain that had been there for almost three
years. Pretty neat!"*

BLOOD TYPE OUTCOME: WEIGHT LOSS AND PAIN RELIEF

"I had seen a rheumatologist for extremely painful arthritis in my hips
and knees. I also had difficulty in other joints, but these were the worst.
After about thirty days of avoiding the foods I should avoid and focusing on those recommended in the Type B Diet, I began to notice significant pain relief. Now, I have virtually no arthritis pain. In addition, I
have lost a significant amount of weight. I had lost weight before, however, and still had the arthritis. The exciting difference to me is the pain-
free state I now enjoy!"

*Self-reported outcomes from the Blood Type Diet web site, www.dadamo.com

HERE'S THE GOOD NEWS. BLOOD TYPE B TYPICALLY HAS fewer risk factors for disease, is more physically fit, and is statistically likely to live a bit longer than the other blood types. By nature, you have a more balanced and "better tempered" immune system. The key is to use the Blood Type Diet and guidelines to minimize the risk factors you *do* have.

Blood Type B is most susceptible to viral and bacterial infections, and these in turn can trigger autoimmune inflammatory responses, often through inactivating complement, or blocking the liver's ability to detoxify normal metabolic waste products. The most common bacteria that produce infections, such as *E. coli*, *Pseudomonas*, and *Klebsiella*, are B-like in appearance, so Blood Type B does not produce antibodies against them. Blood Type B non-secretors are even more prone to these effects. For example, research has demonstrated a direct relationship between being a Type B non-secretor and having an inflammatory response to urinary tract infection (UTI). The reason non-secretors have a higher risk is due to several factors—the inability to prevent adherence of unwanted bacteria, the presence of more binding sites for their attachment, and the tendency to have a more difficult time eliminating bacterial colonization.

Given this propensity, for Blood Type B, the gateway to rheumatoid arthritis and other autoimmune conditions will often be an infection.

The Stress Factor

HIGH STRESS LEVELS ARE implicated in many diseases, and research shows that it plays a role in autoimmune diseases, including arthritis. Stress also has an impact on the severity of the condition.

Under stressful situations, Blood Type B manufactures higher levels of the stress hormone cortisol and has trouble clearing it from the body once the stressful event has passed. That means Blood Type B tends to be in a physiological state of stress, even when external circumstances are not stressful.

For Blood Type B, this dangerous stress response is a consequence

Blood Type B Arthritis-Fighting Food Analysis

ANTI-INFLAMMATORY FOODS	PRO-INFLAMMATORY FOODS
Lamb, goat, mutton	Chicken
Richly oiled cold-water fish	Shellfish
Cultured dairy—e.g., yogurt, kefir	Corn, sesame, sunflower oils
Ghee (clarified butter)	Peanuts and peanut oil
Olive oil	Lentil bean
Flax (linseed) oil	Buckwheat
Onion	Wheat
Maitake mushrooms	Corn
Broccoli	Olives
Blueberries, cherries, elderberries	Tomatoes
Pineapple	Food additives
Ginger	Processed sugar
Licorice root	
Green tea	

of imbalance. When your immune surveillance systems are in balance, which is the way you are meant to be, you are able to block stress, anxiety, and depression, using your powerful gift for relaxation and visualization. Your focus in achieving mind-body integrity needs to be on lowering your cortisol levels and increasing your mental acuity.

A Word to the Wise Type B: Glucosamine and Chondroitin

MANY OF MY PATIENTS have wanted to know if they should take glucosamine and chondroitin. Blood Type B can benefit from taking glucosamine but should avoid chondroitin. Here's why: Glucosamine helps to block inflammation-producing lectins, especially wheat germ lectin, by acting as a decoy. The lectin binds to it instead of binding to your intestinal lining.

Chondroitin is a different matter. If we were to analyze the structure of chondroitin, we would see that it is composed of a repeating sugar, N-acetyl galactosamine. N-acetyl galactosamine is the Blood Type A antigen. Thus, by consuming large amounts of chondroitin, Blood Type B is essentially provoking its immune system with what amounts to an incompatible blood transfusion.

What seems to work best for Blood Type B is a compound called MSM, or methylsufonylmethane. MSM is also called organic sulfur. MSM is a nutrient found in the human diet and the natural diets of virtually all other vertebrates. Although the mechanism of its actions are not totally understood, it is quite safe. Sulfur is widely utilized by the body in the formation of connective tissue and in the product of the antioxidant glutathione, so the benefits of MSM for Blood Type B may be its ability to enhance detoxification, as well.

Blood Type B: The Foods

THE BLOOD TYPE B Arthritis Diet is specifically adapted for the prevention and management of arthritis. A new category, **Super Beneficial,** highlights powerful arthritis-fighting foods for Blood Type B. The **Neutral** category has also been adjusted to de-emphasize foods that are less advantageous for you. Foods designated **Neutral: Allowed Infrequently** should be minimized or avoided entirely.

Food Values

SUPER BENEFICIAL	Foods that are known to have specific disease-fighting qualities for your blood type.
BENEFICIAL	Foods with components that enhance the metabolic, immune, or structural health of you blood type.
NEUTRAL: Allowed Infrequently	Foods that normally have no direct type effect but may impede your progress when consumed regularly.
AVOID	Foods with components that are harmful to your blood type.

Your secretor status can influence your ability to fully digest and metabolize certain foods, so various adjustments in the values are made for non-secretors. If you do not know your secretor type, the odds are that you can safely use the "secretor" values, since the majority of the population (approximately 80 percent) are secretors. However, I urge you to get tested, since the variations are important for non-secretors who want to maximize the effectiveness of the Blood Type Diet.

The food charts are divided into three sections. The top of the chart suggests the average portion size and quantity per week or day, according to secretor status. These recommendations do *not* apply to the category **Neutral: Allowed Infrequently;** those foods should be eaten rarely, if at all. The charts also indicate differences in frequency for some foods, based on ethnic heritage. It has been my experience that this factor has an impact upon the individual's ability to fully digest certain foods. For the purposes of blood type food choices, persons of Hispanic heritage should follow the recommendations for Caucasians, and North American Native peoples should follow the recommendations for Asians.

The middle section of the chart gives the food values. The bottom section lists variants based on secretor status.

For your convenience, we have included a number of product names (Ezekiel bread, Worcestershire sauce, etc.). However, keep in mind that commercial formulations vary among brands and regions. Even though a product may be listed as acceptable for you, always check its ingredients; do not use products that contain **Avoid** ingredients for your blood type. Of course, you may choose to make your own version of commercial products, such as bread and mayonnaise, using ingredients that suit your blood type. There are hundreds of delicious recipes for every blood type available on our Web site (www.dadamo. com) and in the book *Cook Right 4 Your Type: The Practical Kitchen Companion to* Eat Right 4 Your Type.

Meat/Poultry

Blood Type B is able to efficiently metabolize animal protein, but there are limitations that require careful dietary navigation. Chicken, one of the most popular food choices, disagrees with Blood Type B because of a B-specific agglutinin, called a galectin, contained in the organ and muscle meat. This galectin can trigger inflammatory and autoimmune conditions. Turkey does not contain this lectin and can be eaten as an excellent alternative to chicken. The leaner cuts of lamb and mutton should be a part of your diet. They help build muscle and active tissue mass, thus reducing the risk of joint deterioration. Blood Type B non-secretors should increase their weekly intake of meat and poultry.

Limit organ meats if you have gout. They are particularly high sources of purine, which is known to exacerbate that condition.

Choose only the best-quality (preferably free-range), chemical-, antibiotic-, and pesticide-free, low-fat meats and poultry. Grass-fed cattle are far superior to grain-fed.

BLOOD TYPE B: MEAT/POULTRY			
Portion: 4–6 oz (men); 2–5 oz (women and children)			
	African	Caucasian	Asian
Secretor	3–6	2–6	2–5
Non-Secretor	4–7	4–7	4–7
		Times per week	

SUPER BENEFICIAL	BENEFICIAL	NEUTRAL: Allowed Frequently	NEUTRAL: Allowed Infrequently	AVOID
Goat Lamb Mutton	Rabbit Venison	Beef Buffalo Ostrich Pheasant Turkey Veal	Liver (calf)	All commercially processed meats Bacon/Ham/Pork Chicken Cornish hen Duck Goose Grouse Guinea hen Heart (beef)

SUPER BENEFICIAL	BENEFICIAL	NEUTRAL: Allowed Frequently	NEUTRAL: Allowed Infrequently	AVOID
				Horse Partridge Quail Squab Squirrel Sweetbreads Turtle

Special Variants: *Non-Secretor* NEUTRAL (Allowed Frequently): heart (beef), horse, squab, sweetbreads.

Fish/Seafood

Fish and seafood are an excellent source of protein for Blood Type B. Fish is a treasure trove of dense nutrients and is particularly beneficial for non-secretors. Seafood can be an excellent source of docosahexaenoic acid (DHA), a nutrient needed for proper nerve, tissue, and growth function. Richly oiled cold-water fish, such as halibut, mackerel, cod, salmon, and sardines, are especially good arthritis fighters, since they are excellent sources of anti-inflammatory omega-3 fatty acids. Do not waste your money on "farm-raised" fish: They have almost none of these precious oils.

BLOOD TYPE B: FISH/SEAFOOD			
Portion: 4–6 oz (men); 2–5 oz. (women and children)			
	African	Caucasian	Asian
Secretor	4–5	3–5	3–5
Non-Secretor	4–5	4–5	4–5
	Times per week		

SUPER BENEFICIAL	BENEFICIAL	NEUTRAL: Allowed Frequently	NEUTRAL: Allowed Infrequently	AVOID
Cod	Caviar	Abalone	Herring	Anchovy
Halibut	(sturgeon)	Bluefish	(smoked)	Barracuda
Mackerel	Croaker	Bullhead	Salmon	Bass (all)
Salmon	Flounder	Carp	(smoked)	Beluga
Sardine	Grouper	Catfish		Butterfish
	Haddock	Chub		Clam
	Hake	Cusk		Conch
	Harvest	Drum		Crab
	fish	Gray sole		Eel
	Mahi-mahi	Halfmoon		Frog
	Monkfish	fish		Lobster
	Perch	Herring		Mussels
	(ocean)	(fresh/		Octopus
	Pickerel	pickled)		Oysters
	Pike	Mullet		Pollock
	Porgy	Muskel-		Salmon roe
	Shad	lunge		Shrimp
	Sole	Opaleye		Snail (Helix
	Sturgeon	fish		pomatia/
		Orange		escargot)
		roughy		Trout (all)
		Parrot		Yellowtail
		fish		
		Perch		
		(silver/		
		white/		
		yellow)		
		Pompano		
		Red		
		snapper		
		Rosefish		
		Sailfish		
		Scallops		
		Scrod		
		Scup		
		Shark		
		Smelt		
		Snapper		

SUPER BENEFICIAL	BENEFICIAL	NEUTRAL: Allowed Frequently	NEUTRAL: Allowed Infrequently	AVOID
		Squid (calamari) Sucker Sunfish Swordfish Tilapia Tilefish Tuna Weakfish Whitefish Whiting		

Special Variants: *Non-Secretor* BENEFICIAL: carp; Gray sole; NEUTRAL (Allowed Frequently): barracuda, butterfish, caviar (sturgeon), flounder, halibut, pike, salmon, snail (*Helix pomatia*/escargot), sole, yellowtail; AVOID: scallops.

Dairy/Eggs

Dairy—especially cultured dairy products—can be eaten by almost all Blood Type B secretors and to a lesser degree by non-secretors. Cultured dairy, such as yogurt and kefir, is particularly good for Blood Type B; these foods help build a healthy intestinal environment. Ghee (clarified butter) contains beneficial fatty acids believed to promote intestinal balance. Non-secretors should be wary of eating too much cheese, as they are more sensitive to many of the microbial strains in aged cheeses. This sensitivity is greater if you are of African ancestry, but the sensitivity can also be found in Caucasian and Asian populations. Also limit your cheese consumption if you suffer from recurrent infections or allergies, as cheese can trigger inflammation and produce excess mucus. Eggs are a good source of DHA (docosahexaenoil acid) for Blood Type B and can be an integral part of your protein requirement. Try to find dairy products that are both hormone-free and organic.

BLOOD TYPE B: EGGS			
Portion: 1 egg			
	African	Caucasian	Asian
Secretor	3–4	3–4	3–4
Non-Secretor	5–6	5–6	5–6
		Times per week	

BLOOD TYPE B: MILK AND YOGURT			
Portion: 4–6 oz (men); 2–5 oz (women and children)			
	African	Caucasian	Asian
Secretor	3–5	3–4	3–4
Non-Secretor	1–3	2–4	1–3
		Times per week	

BLOOD TYPE B: CHEESE			
Portion: 3 oz (men); 2 oz (women and children)			
	African	Caucasian	Asian
Secretor	3–4	3–5	3–4
Non-Secretor	1–4	1–4	1–4
		Times per week	

SUPER BENEFICIAL	BENEFICIAL	NEUTRAL: Allowed Frequently	NEUTRAL: Allowed Infrequently	AVOID
Ghee (clarified butter)	Cottage cheese	Camembert	Brie	American cheese
Kefir	Farmer cheese	Casein	Butter	Blue cheese
Yogurt	Feta	Cream cheese	Buttermilk	Egg (duck/ goose/ quail)
	Goat cheese	Edam	Cheddar	Ice cream
	Milk (cow/ goat)	Egg (chicken)	Colby	String cheese
	Mozzarella	Emmenthal	Half-and- half	
	Paneer	Gouda	Jarlsberg	
	Ricotta	Gruyère	Monterey Jack	
		Neufchâtel	Muenster	
		Parmesan	Sherbet	
			Sour cream	

SUPER BENEFICIAL	BENEFICIAL	NEUTRAL: Allowed Frequently	NEUTRAL: Allowed Infrequently	AVOID
		Provolone Quark	Swiss cheese Whey	

Special Variants: *Non-Secretor* NEUTRAL (Allowed Frequently): cottage cheese, milk (cow); AVOID: Camembert, cheddar, Emmenthal, Jarlsberg, Monterey Jack, Muenster, Parmesan, provolone, Swiss cheese.

Oils

Blood Type B does best on monounsaturated oils and oils rich in omega series fatty acids. Olive oil fits the bill in both regards. Constituents in olive oil, such as flavonoids, squalenes, and polyphenols, act as powerful antioxidants. Use it as your primary cooking oil.

Make it a point to avoid sesame, sunflower, and corn oils, which can contain immunoreactive proteins that impair Blood Type B digestion. These oils can interfere with proper immune function and stimulate the inflammatory response.

BLOOD TYPE B: OILS			
Portion: 1 tblsp			
	African	Caucasian	Asian
Secretor	5–8	5–8	5–8
Non-Secretor	3–5	3–7	3–6
		Times per week	

SUPER BENEFICIAL	BENEFICIAL	NEUTRAL: Allowed Frequently	NEUTRAL: Allowed Infrequently	AVOID
Flax (lin-seed) Olive		Almond Black currant seed Cod liver Evening primrose Walnut	Wheat germ	Avocado Borage seed Canola Castor Coconut Corn Cottonseed Peanut Safflower Sesame Soy Sunflower

Special Variants: *Non-Secretor* BENEFICIAL: black currant seed, walnut.

Nuts and Seeds

Nuts and seeds can be an important secondary source of protein for Blood Type B. Laboratory research has identified at least five natural phytochemicals in nuts that regulate the immune system and act as antioxidants. Black walnuts are also SUPER BENEFICIAL. They are one of the best plant sources of omega-3 fatty acids. Walnuts are also highly effective in inhibiting gastrointestinal toxicity because they minimize the production of chemicals called polyamines.

As with other aspects of the Blood Type B Diet plan, there are some idiosyncratic elements to the choice of seeds and nuts: Several, such as sunflower and sesame, have B-agglutinating lectins and should be avoided.

BLOOD TYPE B: NUTS AND SEEDS			
Portion: Whole (handful); Nut Butters (2 tblsp)			
	African	Caucasian	Asian
Secretor	4–7	4–7	4–7
Non-Secretor	5–7	5–7	5–7
		Times per week	

SUPER BENEFICIAL	BENEFICIAL	NEUTRAL: Allowed Frequently	NEUTRAL: Allowed Infrequently	AVOID
Walnut (black)		Almond Almond butter Almond cheese Almond milk Beechnut Brazil nut Butternut Chestnut Hickory Flax (linseed) Walnut (English)	Litchi Macadamia Pecan	Cashew Filbert (hazelnut) Peanut Peanut butter Pignolia (pine nut) Pistachio Poppy seed Pumpkin seed Safflower seed Sesame butter (tahini) Sesame seed Sunflower butter Sunflower seed

Special Variants: *Non-Secretor* NEUTRAL (Allowed Frequently): pumpkin seed.

Beans and Legumes

Blood Type B can do well on proteins found in many beans and legumes, although this food category does contain more than a few beans with problematic lectins. Soy beans should be minimized, and related soy products should be avoided, as they are rich in a class of enzymes that can interact negatively with the B antigen. Several beans, such as mung beans, contain B-agglutinating lectins and should be avoided. These lectins are associated with inflammation.

BLOOD TYPE B: BEANS AND LEGUMES			
Portion: 1 cup (cooked)			
	African	**Caucasian**	**Asian**
Secretor	5–7	5–7	5–7
Non-Secretor	3–5	3–5	3–5
	Times per week		

SUPER BENEFICIAL	BENEFICIAL	NEUTRAL: Allowed Frequently	NEUTRAL: Allowed Infrequently	AVOID
	Kidney bean Lima bean Navy bean	Bean (green/ snap/ string) Cannellini bean Copper bean Fava (broad) bean Jicama bean Northern bean Pea (green/ pod/ snow) Soy bean Tamarind bean White bean		Adzuki bean Black bean Black-eyed pea Garbanzo (chickpea) Lentil (all) Miso Mung bean/ sprout Pinto bean Soy cheese Soy milk Tempeh Tofu

Special Variants: *Non-Secretor* NEUTRAL (Allowed Frequently): kidney bean, lima bean, navy bean; AVOID: soy bean.

Grains and Starches

Grains are a leading factor in triggering inflammatory and autoimmune conditions in Blood Type B. The wheat agglutinin is particularly harmful, as is the lectin in corn. Non-secretors have an even greater sensitivity. Sprouted grains, such as Essene (manna) bread, are the exception. Sprouting makes the grains less reactive to the Type B immune system.

BLOOD TYPE B: GRAINS AND STARCHES			
Portion: ½ cup dry (grains or pastas); 1 muffin; 2 slices of bread			
	African	Caucasian	Asian
Secretor	5–7	5–9	5–9
Non-Secretor	3–5	3–5	3–5
			Times per week

SUPER BENEFICIAL	BENEFICIAL	NEUTRAL: Allowed Frequently	NEUTRAL: Allowed Infrequently	AVOID
	Essene bread (manna) Ezekiel bread Millet Oat bran Oat flour Oatmeal Rice bran Rice cake Rice milk Spelt (whole)	Barley Quinoa Rice (whole) Spelt flour/ products 100% sprouted grain products (except Essene)	Rice flour Soy flour/ products Wheat (re-fined/un-bleached) Wheat (se-molina) Wheat (white flour)	Amaranth Buckwheat Cornmeal Couscous Grits Kamut Popcorn Potato Rice (wild) Rye (whole) Rye flour/ products Soba noodles (100% buckwheat) Sorghum Tapioca Teff

SUPER BENEFICIAL	BENEFICIAL	NEUTRAL: Allowed Frequently	NEUTRAL: Allowed Infrequently	AVOID
				Wheat (whole) Wheat bran Wheat germ

Special Variants: *Non-Secretor* NEUTRAL (Allowed Frequently): amaranth, Ezekiel oat (all), rice (wild), sorghum, spelt (whole), tapioca; AVOID: wheat.

Vegetables

Vegetables can be your first line of defense against chronic disease. They provide a rich source of antioxidants and fiber and are essential to intestinal health. Blood Type B SUPER BENEFICIALS include onions and garlic, which are high in quercetin, a flavonoid with potent anti-inflammatory properties, and other antioxidants that decrease oxidative stress and increase glutathione, which protects cells. Onions and garlic are also rich sources of diallyl sulfide, which detoxifies carcinogens. Broccoli contains allyl methyl trisulfide and dithiolthiones, which increase the activity of enzymes involved in detoxification. This is critical for Blood Type Bs who want to control inflammation. Sweet potatoes are rich in vitamins A and B_6, which stabilize immune function. Cabbage, Brussels sprouts, and cauliflower positively influence Blood Type B's immune system, reducing susceptibility to viruses. Maitake and shiitake mushrooms are powerful antiviral agents as well.

Tomatoes contain a lectin that reacts with the saliva and digestive juices of Blood Type B secretors, although it does not appear to react with non-secretors. Corn has B-agglutinating activity and should be avoided.

An item's value also applies to its juice, unless otherwise noted.

BLOOD TYPE B: VEGETABLES			
Portion: 1 cup, prepared (cooked or raw)			
	African	**Caucasian**	**Asian**
Secretor Super/ Beneficials	Unlimited	Unlimited	Unlimited
Secretor Neutrals	2–5	2–5	2–5
Non-Secretor Super/ Beneficials	Unlimited	Unlimited	Unlimited
Non-Secretor Neutrals	2–3	2–3	2–3
			Times per day

SUPER BENEFICIAL	BENEFICIAL	NEUTRAL: Allowed Frequently	NEUTRAL: Allowed Infrequently	AVOID
Broccoli Brussels sprouts Cabbage Cabbage (juice)* Cauliflower Garlic Mushroom (maitake/ shiitake) Onion (all) Potato (sweet)	Beet Beet greens Carrot Collards Eggplant Kale Mushroom (silver dollar) Mustard greens Parsnip Peppers (all) Yam	Alfalfa sprouts Arugula Asparagus Asparagus pea Bamboo shoots Bok choy Carrot (juice) Celeriac Celery Chicory Cucumber Daikon radish Dandelion Endive Escarole Fennel Fiddlehead fern Horse-radish	Pickle (in brine or vine-gar)	Aloe Artichoke Corn Olive (all) Pumpkin Radish/ sprouts Rhubarb Tomato

SUPER BENEFICIAL	BENEFICIAL	NEUTRAL: Allowed Frequently	NEUTRAL: Allowed Infrequently	AVOID
		Kohlrabi		
		Leek		
		Lettuce (all)		
		Mushroom (abalone/ enoki/ oyster/ porto- bello/ straw/ tree ear)		
		Okra		
		Oyster plant		
		Poi		
		Radicchio		
		Rappini (broccoli rabe)		
		Rutabaga		
		Scallion		
		Seaweeds		
		Shallot		
		Spinach		
		Squash (all)		
		Swiss chard		
		Taro		
		Turnip		
		Water chestnut		
		Watercress		
		Yucca		
		Zucchini		

Special Variants: *Non-Secretor* BENEFICIAL: okra; NEUTRAL (Allowed Frequently): artichoke, cabbage, cabbage (juice),* eggplant, mushroom (silver dollar), peppers (all), pumpkin, tomato; AVOID: potato.

*To obtain the benefits of cabbage juice, it must be consumed within one minute of juicing.

Fruits and Fruit Juices

Fruits are rich in antioxidants. Many, such as blueberries, elderberries, cherries, and blackberries, are high in anthocyanins, which enhance collagen integrity. Pineapple contains bromelain, a powerful enzyme that has an anti-inflammatory effect on muscle and tissue. Pineapple is also a good source of vitamin C, a deficiency of which is seen in many cases of arthritis. Red grapefruit and watermelon supply the antioxidant lycopene, in lieu of using tomatoes. Plums and prunes are high in the phytonutrients neochlorogenic acid and chlorogenic acid. These substances are classified as phenols, and their function as antioxidants has been well documented. Cranberries are SUPER BENEFICIAL for Blood Type B individuals, especially non-secretors, who have a higher than average risk for urinary tract infections.

An item's value also applies to its juice, unless otherwise noted.

BLOOD TYPE B: FRUITS AND FRUIT JUICES			
Portion: 1 cup			
	African	Caucasian	Asian
Secretor	2–4	3–5	3–5
Non-Secretor	2–3	2–3	2–3
			Times per day

SUPER BENEFICIAL	BENEFICIAL	NEUTRAL: Allowed Frequently	NEUTRAL: Allowed Infrequently	AVOID
Blackberry	Banana	Apple	Apricot	Avocado
Blueberry	Grape (all)	Boysenberry	Asian	Bitter melon
Cherry	Papaya	Canang	pear	Coconut
Cranberry		melon	Breadfruit	Persimmon
Elderberry		Casaba	Cantaloupe	Pome-
Grapefruit		melon	Currant	granate
(red)		Christmas	Date	Prickly pear
Guava		melon	Fig (fresh/	Star fruit
Pineapple		Crenshaw	dried)	(carambola)
Plum (all)		melon		

SUPER BENEFICIAL	BENEFICIAL	NEUTRAL: Allowed Frequently	NEUTRAL: Allowed Infrequently	AVOID
Water-melon		Dewberry Gooseberry Grapefruit (white) Kiwi Kumquat Lemon Lime Loganberry Mango Mulberry Muskmelon Nectarine Orange Peach Pear Persian melon Plantain Prune Quince Raspberry Sago palm Spanish melon Strawberry Tangerine Youngberry	Honeydew melon Raisin	

Special Variants: *Non-Secretor* BENEFICIAL: boysenberry, currant, fig (dried/fresh), raspberry; NEUTRAL (Allowed Frequently): banana, grapefruit (red); AVOID: cantaloupe, honeydew melon.

Spices/Condiments/Sweeteners

Many spices are known to have anti-inflammatory properties. The common cooking spices—rosemary, thyme, and oregano—are powerful antioxidants that exert anti-inflammatory effects. Turmeric and garlic are also anti-inflammatory. Ginger inhibits the production of COX-2, an enzyme that triggers the inflammatory response. Parsley contains quercetin, which is anti-inflammatory. Licorice root provides antiviral support.

Many common food additives, such as guar gum and carrageenan, enhance the effects of lectins found in other foods and should be avoided. Use caution when using prepared condiments. Often they contain wheat, which is a primary factor in the development of arthritis and other inflammatory conditions.

SUPER BENEFICIAL	BENEFICIAL	NEUTRAL: Allowed Frequently	NEUTRAL: Allowed Infrequently	AVOID
Ginger	Dill	Anise	Agar	Allspice
Licorice	Horse-	Apple	Arrowroot	Almond
root*	radish	pectin	Chocolate	extract
Oregano	Molasses	Basil	Fructose	Aspartame
Pepper	(black-	Bay leaf	Honey	Barley malt
(cayenne)	strap)	Bergamot	Maple	Carrageenan
Rosemary	Parsley	Caper	syrup	Cinnamon
Thyme	Tarragon	Caraway	Mayonnaise	Cornstarch
Turmeric		Cardamom	Molasses	Corn syrup
		Carob	Pickles (all)	Dextrose
		Chervil	Rice syrup	Gelatin (ex-
		Chili pow-	Sugar	cept veg-
		der	(brown/	sourced)
		Chive	white)	Guarana
		Cilantro	Tamari	Gums (aca-
		(coriander	(wheat-	cia/Arabic/
		leaf)	free)	guar)
		Clove	Vinegar (all)	Invert sugar
		Coriander		Juniper

SUPER BENEFICIAL	BENEFICIAL	NEUTRAL: Allowed Frequently	NEUTRAL: Allowed Infrequently	AVOID
		Cream of tartar	Yeast (baker's/ brewer's)	Ketchup
		Cumin		Maltodextrin
		Garlic		MSG
		Lecithin		Pepper
		Mace		(black/
		Marjoram		white)
		Mint (all)		Pickle
		Mustard		(relish)
		(dry)		Soy sauce
		Nutmeg		Stevia
		Paprika		Sucanat
		Pepper		Tapioca
		(pepper-		Worcester-
		corn/red		shire sauce
		flakes)		
		Saffron		
		Sage		
		Savory		
		Sea salt		
		Seaweeds		
		Senna		
		Tamarind		
		Vanilla		
		Wintergreen		

Special Variants: *Non-Secretor* BENEFICIAL: yeast (brewer's); NEUTRAL (Allowed Frequently): dill, stevia, tarragon; AVOID: agar, fructose, pickle (relish), sugar (brown/white).

*Do not use if you have high blood pressure.

Herbal Teas

Several herbal teas can be SUPER BENEFICIAL arthritis fighters for Blood Type B. Ginger contains pungent phenolic substances with pronounced antioxidative and anti-inflammatory activities. Sage is rich in rosmarinic acid, which acts to reduce inflammatory responses by altering the concentrations of inflammatory messaging molecules. The leaves and stems of the sage plant contain antioxidant enzymes, including superoxide dismutase (SOD) and peroxidase. When combined, these three components of sage—flavonoids, phenolic acids, and oxygen-handling enzymes—give it a unique capacity for stabilizing oxygen-related metabolism and preventing oxygen-based damage to the cells. Licorice root tea provides antiviral support for Blood Type B.

SUPER BENEFICIAL	BENEFICIAL	NEUTRAL: Allowed Frequently	NEUTRAL: Allowed Infrequently	AVOID
Ginger	Ginseng	Alfalfa		Aloe
Licorice	Parsley	Burdock		Coltsfoot
root*	Peppermint	Catnip		Corn silk
Sage	Raspberry	Chamomile		Fenugreek
	leaf	Chickweed		Gentian
	Rosehip	Dandelion		Hops
		Dong quai		Linden
		Echinacea		Mullein
		Elder		Red clover
		Goldenseal		Rhubarb
		Hawthorn		Shepherd's
		Horehound		purse
		Mulberry		Skullcap
		Rosemary		
		Sarsaparilla		
		Senna		
		Slippery		
		elm		
		Spearmint		
		St. John's		
		wort		
		Strawberry		
		leaf		
		Thyme		
		Valerian		
		Vervain		
		White birch		

SUPER BENEFICIAL	BENEFICIAL	NEUTRAL: Allowed Frequently	NEUTRAL: Allowed Infrequently	AVOID
		White oak bark Yarrow Yellow dock		
Special Variants: None				

*Do not use if you have high blood pressure.

Miscellaneous Beverages

Green tea should be part of every Blood Type B's health plan. It contains polyphenols, which enhance gastrointestinal health. It also inhibits TNF-alpha gene expression. TNF-alpha is known to be a central mediator in chronic inflammatory diseases such as rheumatoid arthritis and multiple sclerosis. Avoid or limit alcohol to an occasional glass of red wine. Alcohol can exacerbate autoimmune inflammatory conditions and may be a factor in the development of some forms of arthritis, such as gout. Avoid or limit alcohol to an occasional glass of red wine. If you are a heavy coffee drinker, reduce your intake or eliminate it altogether.

SUPER BENEFICIAL	BENEFICIAL	NEUTRAL: Allowed Frequently	NEUTRAL: Allowed Infrequently	AVOID
Tea (green)		Wine (red/ white)	Beer	Liquor
			Coffee (reg/decaf)	Seltzer Soda (club)
			Tea, black (reg/decaf)	Soda (cola/ diet/misc.)
Special Variants: *Non-Secretor* BENEFICIAL: wine (red/white); NEUTRAL (Allowed Frequently): seltzer, soda (club); AVOID: coffee (reg/decaf), tea (black: reg/decaf).				

Supplements

THE BLOOD TYPE B DIET offers abundant quantities of important nutrients, such as protein and iron. It is important to get as many nutrients as possible from fresh foods and use supplements only to fill in the minor deficiencies in your diet. The following supplement protocols are designed for Blood Type B individuals who are suffering from arthritis or related autoimmune conditions.

Note: If you are being treated for a medical condition, consult your doctor before taking any supplements.

Blood Type B: Anti-Inflammatory Protocol

Use this protocol for 12 weeks to prevent and minimize inflammatory conditions, while balancing immune function.		
SUPPLEMENT	**ACTION**	**DOSAGE**
MSM (methylsulfonyl-methane)	Promotes joint and pulmonary health	500 mg, twice daily
Niacin (vitamin B$_3$)*	Promotes healthy digestion and metabolism	50 mg, 2 capsules daily
Magnesium	Vital nutrient	300–500 mg daily
Maitake extract (*Grifola frondosa*)	Antiviral agent	500 mg, twice daily
Cat's claw (*Uncaria tomentosa*)	Acts as an anti-inflammatory	500 mg, twice daily
Jiaogulan (*Gynostemma penta phylum*)	Acts as an anti-inflammatory	60 mg gynostemma whole glucosides, twice daily
Quercetin	Has anti-inflammatory effects	500 mg, twice daily, away from food
Larch arabino-galactan (*Larix officinalis*)	Promotes digestive and intestinal health	1 tablespoon, twice daily, in juice or water

* Do not exceed recommended dosage.

Blood Type B: Arthritis Pain Relief Adjunct

Use this protocol for 4 weeks to reduce pain associated with joint disease.

SUPPLEMENT	ACTION	DOSAGE
Cayenne pepper (*Capsicum* sp.)	Arthritis pain relief	300 mg, 1–2 capsules with meals or topically in cream
Bromelain (pineapple enzyme)	Has antioxidant and anti-inflammatory properties	500 mg, 1–3 capsules daily with meals, gradually decreasing dose and frequency as symptoms improve

Blood Type B: Joint Repair Adjunct

Use this protocol for 4 weeks to promote healing and improve joint integrity.

SUPPLEMENT	ACTION	DOSAGE
Glucosamine sulfate	Enables joint repair	500 mg, 2–3 capsules daily, away from food
S-adenosylmethione (SAMe)*	Stimulates collagen production	400 mg, 1–2 capsules daily
Vitamin C (rose hips or acerola cherry)	Promotes healing	250 mg, twice daily

* Do not use if you have Parkinson's disease.

Blood Type B: Surgery Recovery Adjunct

When surgery is scheduled, add this protocol for 2 weeks before surgery and 2 weeks after.

SUPPLEMENT	ACTION	DOSAGE
Rehmannia root) (*Rehmannia glutinosa*)	Promotes healing of injured bones; aids blood clotting	200 mg, 1 capsule daily

SUPPLEMENT	ACTION	DOSAGE
White atractylodes (*Atractylodis macrocephalae*)	Liver protective; digestive secretion stimulant	250 mg, 1 capsule daily
L-arginine	Immune enhancement; promotes healing; boosts nitric oxide	250 mg, twice daily

The Exercise Component

THE BEST WISDOM OF BOTH conventional and naturopathic medicine is that regular exercise, including aerobic activity and weights, is essential to fighting arthritis and autoimmune diseases. It may seem counterintuitive, since arthritis makes movement difficult and often painful. However, studies consistently show that aerobic exercise can reduce joint swelling. Strength training builds muscle, helping to support and protect joints affected by arthritis. Physical exercise also promotes lean muscle mass and reduces weight, thus lightening the load on stressed joints.

For Blood Type B, stress regulation and overall fitness are achieved with a balance of moderate aerobic activity and mentally soothing, stress-reducing exercises. Below is a list of exercises for Blood Type B.

EXERCISE	DURATION	FREQUENCY
Tennis	45–60 minutes	2–3 x week
Martial arts	30–60 minutes	2–3 x week
Cycling	45–60 minutes	2–3 x week
Hiking	30–60 minutes	2–3 x week
Golf (no cart!)	60–90 minutes	2–3 x week
Running or brisk walking	40–50 minutes	2–3 x week
Pilates	40–50 minutes	2–3 x week
Swimming	45 minutes	2–3 x week
Yoga	40–50 minutes	1–2 x week
T'ai Chi	40–50 minutes	1–2 x week

3 Steps to Effective Exercise

1. Warm up with stretching and flexibility moves before you start your aerobic exercise.
2. To achieve maximum cardiovascular benefits, work toward an elevated heart rate that is about 70 percent of your capacity. Once you reach the elevated rate, continue exercising to maintain that rate for twenty to thirty minutes. To calculate your maximum heart rate and performance level:
   - Subtract your age from 220.
   - Multiply the difference by .70 (or .60 if you are over age sixty). This is the high end of your performance.
   - Multiply the remainder by .50. This is the low end of your performance.
3. Finish each aerobic session with at least a five-minute cooldown of stretching and relaxation moves.

Getting Started: The First Month

IF YOU ARE NEW to the Blood Type Diet, the following guidelines will introduce you to the Blood Type B regimen over a period of one month. Follow these recommendations as closely as possible, using a journal to record your personal experiences with the diet. In addition to factors that are measurable in laboratory tests, take the time to note changes in your energy levels, pain levels, sleep patterns, digestion, and overall well-being.

Blood Type B Arthritis Diet Checklist

Eat small to moderate portions of high-quality, lean, organic ☐ meat (especially goat, lamb, and mutton) several times a week for strength, energy, and digestive health. Meat should be prepared medium to rare for the best health effects. If you charbroil, or cook meat well-done, use a marinade composed of beneficial ingredients, such as cherry juice, spices, and herbs.

Include regular portions of richly oiled cold-water fish. Fish ☐ oils can help counter inflammatory conditions and balance immune activity.

If you are not accustomed to eating dairy products, introduce ☐ them gradually, after you have been on the diet for Blood Type B for several weeks. Begin with cultured dairy foods, such as yogurt and kefir, which are more easily tolerated.

Eliminate wheat and wheat-based products from your diet. ☐ They are the primary culprits in many arthritic and auto-immune diseases.

Eat lots of BENEFICIAL fruits and vegetables. ☐

If you need a daily dose of caffeine, replace coffee with green ☐ tea. It isn't acidic and has substantially less caffeine than a cup of coffee.

Use BENEFICIAL and NEUTRAL nuts and dried fruits for snacks. ☐

Avoid foods that are Type B red flags, especially chicken, corn, ☐ buckwheat, peanuts, lentils, and potatoes.

Week 1

Blood Type Diet and Supplements

- Eliminate your most harmful AVOID foods—chicken, corn, and buckwheat. The lectins in these foods can trigger inflammation.

- Avoid wheat if you have arthritis.

- Include your most important BENEFICIAL foods on a regular schedule throughout the week. For example, have lean red meat 5 times, and omega-3-rich fish 3 to 4 times, with lots of BENEFICIAL vegetables and fruit.

- Incorporate at least 1 SUPER BENEFICIAL food into your daily diet. For example, have a handful of walnuts as a snack, or eat yogurt mixed with berries for lunch.

- If you're a coffee drinker, begin to wean yourself by cutting your daily consumption in half, substituting green tea or a SUPER BENEFICIAL herbal tea.

Exercise Regimen

- Plan to exercise at least 4 days this week, for 45 minutes each day.

  2–3 days: aerobic activity

  1–2 days: yoga or T'ai Chi

- If you have joint impairment, start slowly and gradually increase your duration and intensity of activity. The important factor is consistency. Just do it—as much as you're able.

- Use your journal to detail the time, activity, distance, and amount of weight. Note the number of repetitions for each exercise.

▪ WEEK 1 SUCCESS STRATEGY ▪
Infection Busters

With an increased susceptibility to infection, which can serve as a gateway to inflammatory conditions, Blood Type B individuals must stay vigilant. Here are some tips:

- Eat plenty of cultured dairy foods to encourage a healthy intestinal environment and a balanced urinary tract.

- Eat fruits friendly to your urinary tract. Drink organic cranberry or blueberry juice every day.

- Keep your kitchen bacteria-free: Clean preparation areas thoroughly, use disposable cloths and sponges, and wash your hands often. Use separate cutting boards for meat and produce.

- Cook meat thoroughly.

- Purchase disposable masks to cover your mouth and nose on airplanes, especially during the cold and flu season. Curb your embarrassment!

Week 2

Blood Type Diet and Supplements

- Begin to eliminate the next level of AVOID foods—seeds, beans, and legumes that have negative lectin activity.

- Eat at least 2 to 3 BENEFICIAL animal proteins every day, such as lamb, yogurt, or seafood.

- Initially, it is best to avoid foods on the list NEUTRAL: Allowed Infrequently.

- Continue to incorporate SUPER BENEFICIAL foods into your daily diet.

- If you're a coffee drinker, continue to cut your coffee intake, replacing it with green tea or SUPER BENEFICIAL herbal teas.

Exercise Regimen

- Continue to exercise at least 4 days this week for 45 minutes each day.

  2–3 days: aerobic activity

  1–2 days: yoga or T'ai Chi

- If your work is sedentary, get in the habit of taking a couple of "movement" breaks during the day. Walk around the block or up and down stairs. Movement will help maintain joint flexibility.

▪ WEEK 2 SUCCESS STRATEGY ▪
Boost Your Liver Function

A castor oil pack can stimulate the liver, relieve pain, increase lymphatic circulation, reduce inflammation, and improve digestion.

HOW TO MAKE A CASTOR OIL PACK

MATERIALS

- Three layers of dye-free wool or cotton flannel large enough to cover the affected area
- Castor oil
- Plastic wrap cut 1–2" larger than the flannel (can be cut from a plastic bag)
- Hot water bottle
- Container with lid
- Old clothes and sheets. Castor oil will stain clothing and bedding.

METHOD

1. Place the flannel in the container. Soak it in castor oil so that it is saturated, but not dripping.
2. Place the pack over the affected body part.
3. Cover with plastic.
4. Place the hot water bottle over the pack. Leave it on for 45–60 minutes. Rest while the pack is in place.
5. After removing the pack, cleanse the area with a diluted solution of water and baking soda.
6. Store the pack in the covered container in the refrigerator. Each pack may be reused 25–30 times.

WHERE TO PLACE THE CASTOR OIL PACK

A castor oil pack can be placed on the following body regions:

- The right side of the abdomen to stimulate the liver. Castor oil packs are often recommended as part of a liver detox program.
- Inflamed and swollen joints, bursitis, and muscle strains.
- The abdomen to relieve constipation and other digestive disorders.
- The lower abdomen in cases of menstrual irregularities and uterine and ovarian cysts.

SAFETY PRECAUTIONS

Castor oil should not be taken internally. It should not be applied to broken skin, or used during pregnancy, breastfeeding, or during menstrual flow.

FREQUENCY OF USE

It is generally recommended that a castor oil pack be used for 3 to 7 days in a week to treat a health condition or for detoxification.

Week 3

Blood Type Diet and Supplements

- When you plan your meals for week 3, choose BENEFICIAL foods to replace NEUTRAL foods whenever possible. For example, choose lamb over beef, or blueberries over an apple.
- Eliminate all remaining AVOID foods.
- Liberally incorporate SUPER BENEFICIAL foods into your daily diet.

Exercise Regimen

- Continue to exercise at least 4 days this week, for 45 minutes each day.

  2–3 days: aerobic activity

  1–2 days: yoga or Tai Chi

■ WEEK 3 SUCCESS STRATEGY ■
The B Health Cocktail

Flaxseeds are so beneficial to your health, you may want to drink this specially formulated "Membrane Fluidizer Cocktail" every day.

1 tablespoon flaxseed (linseed) oil
1 tablespoon high-quality lecithin granules
6–8 ounces of fruit juice

Shake well and drink.

Week 4

Blood Type Diet and Supplements

- Continue at the week 3 level, focusing on BENEFICIAL and SUPER BENEFICIAL foods.
- Evaluate the first 4 weeks and make adjustments.

Exercise Regimen

- Continue at the week 3 level.
- Review your progress, noting in your journal improvements in strength and flexibility. Determine which exercise regimen has worked for you, including time of day, setting, and activity level.

■ WEEK 4 SUCCESS STRATEGY ■
Tips for Type B Seniors

- A daily regimen of stretching, yoga, and meditation will lower cortisol levels and increase your mental acuity. High cortisol levels have been linked to inflammatory conditions.

- Be especially careful with hygiene and safe food preparation. Type Bs are particularly vulnerable to bacterial infections. If your sense of smell has declined and you have trouble judging freshness by smell, try to have a younger friend or relative accompany you grocery shopping.

- Maintaining a circadian rhythm—important for control of cortisol levels—can be difficult for seniors. Overall, elderly people tend to have more problems with interrupted sleep and insomnia. Ask your doctor about taking supplements of vitamin B_{12} or melatonin.

- Bowel elimination is important for proper detoxification, and most seniors suffer from chronic constipation. Make sure that you are getting plenty of SUPER BENEFICIAL and BENEFICIAL fruits and vegetables. If necessary, take 1000 mg. of magnesium citrate daily with plenty of water to keep your intestines toned and moving.

A Final Word

IN SUMMARY, the secret to fighting arthritis with the Blood Type B Diet involves:

1. Increasing fitness and active tissue mass by adhering to a high-protein diet that includes BENEFICIAL meat, seafood, and dairy.

2. Minimizing the consumption of pro-inflammatory lectins, most abundant in grains such as wheat, buckwheat, and corn.

3. Enhancing detoxification and elimination to increase liver efficiency and inhibit infectious agents.
4. Using supplements intelligently to block the effects of pro-inflammatory lectins, aid detoxification, provide antioxidant support, and protect delicate nerve tissues from destruction.

SEVEN

Blood Type

AB

BLOOD TYPE AB DIET OUTCOME: RESTORED TO BALANCE
"I've stopped snoring, and my arthritis has improved dramatically. If I
do go off the diet, my skin breaks out, almost instantly. I see an acupuncturist, and she says my pulses are better than they have been in the last
seven years."*

BLOOD TYPE AB DIET OUTCOME: RESULTS WIN A CONVERT
"My osteoarthritis is gradually improving and the gastric/elimination
problems which I suffered from after a lifetime of corn and chicken
(which I no longer eat) are just about non-existent. Needless to say, I
make converts wherever I go."

*Self-reported outcomes from the Blood Type Diet web site, www.dadamo.com

B LOOD TYPE AB SEEMS TO BE A BLENDING OF THE A AND B
risk factors for arthritis, with some unique factors that result from
the absence of any opposing blood type antibodies. Like Blood Type A,
the Type AB path to arthritis involves the overstimulation of adhesion

molecules (selectins) on the blood vessel walls, which allows excessive white blood cell migration into the tissues and triggers inflammation.

Like Blood Type B, Type AB is susceptible to viral and bacterial infections, and these in turn can trigger autoimmune inflammatory responses, often through inactivating complement or blocking the liver's ability to detoxify normal metabolic waste products.

Heart Attack Alert

New information about the connection between arthritis and an increased risk of heart attack has special importance for Blood Type AB women. Researchers at the Brigham and Women's Hospital found that women with rheumatoid arthritis had twice the risk of heart attack compared to those without it. Those who had the joint condition for at

Blood Type AB Arthritis-Fighting Food Analysis

ANTI-INFLAMMATORY FOODS	PRO-INFLAMMATORY FOODS
Soy foods	Chicken
Richly oiled cold-water fish	Corn and corn products
Cultured dairy—e.g., eggs yogurt, kefir	Buckwheat
Olive oil	Sesame, sunflower oils and seeds
Flax (linseed) oil	Kidney, lima beans
Walnuts	Bell peppers
Broccoli	Banana
Cauliflower	Coffee
Tomatoes	Food additives
Onion and garlic	Processed sugar
Blueberries, cherries, elderberries	
Grape juice	
Turmeric	
Green tea	

least ten years faced triple the heart attack risks of nonsufferers. There is plenty of evidence that Blood Type AB individuals who are overweight, have high cholesterol, and are diabetic place themselves at grave risk for heart attack. Now we see that there is an arthritis connection as well. All the more reason to eat the right diet for your type.

Glucosamine-Chondroitin and Blood Type AB

SINCE THE INTRODUCTION of the "arthritis cure," many of my patients have wanted to know if they should take glucosamine and chondroitin. I have found that Blood Type AB individuals can effectively use these supplements when they do so in conjunction with the Blood Type Diet.

Glucosamine helps to block inflammation-producing lectins, especially wheat germ lectin, by acting as a decoy. The lectin binds to it instead of binding to the intestinal lining.

While chondroitin is not recommended for every blood type, it provides special advantages for Blood Type AB. Here's why: If we were to analyze the structure of chondroitin, we would see that it is composed of a repeating sugar, N-acetyl galactosamine. N-acetyl galactosamine is the Blood Type A antigen. Thus, by consuming chondroitin, Blood Types A and AB can add a supportive element to your fight against arthritis.

A very good supplement for Blood Type AB is MSM, or methyl-sulfonylmethane. MSM is also called organic sulfur. MSM is a nutrient found in the human diet and the natural diets of virtually all other vertebrates. Although the mechanism of its actions are not totally understood, it is quite safe. Sulfur is widely utilized by the body in the formation of connective tissue and in the production of the antioxidant glutathione, so the benefits of MSM for Blood Type AB may be its ability to enhance detoxification, as well.

Ginger is also a very good supplement for Blood Type AB. Research suggests that ginger root inhibits production of prostaglandins and leukotrienes, which are involved in pain and inflammation. In an uncontrolled 1992 Danish study, fifty-six patients who had either rheumatoid arthritis, osteoarthritis, or muscular discomfort were given powdered ginger. All of those with musculoskeletal pain and three-forths of those with osteoarthritis or rheumatoid arthritis reported varying degrees of pain relief and no side effects, even among those who took the ginger for more than two years. Look for the brands that feature standardized extracts. "Gingerall," by Enzymatic Therapies, is a good product. It is standardized to contain 20 percent total pungent compounds, calculated as 6-gingerol and 6-shogaol.

Blood Type AB: The Foods

THE BLOOD TYPE AB Arthritis Diet is specifically adapted for the prevention and management of arthritis. A new category, **Super Beneficial,** highlights powerful arthritis-fighting foods for Blood Type AB. The **Neutral** category has also been adjusted to de-emphasize foods that are less advantageous for you. Foods designated **Neutral: Allowed Infrequently** should be minimized or avoided entirely.

Food Values

SUPER BENEFICIAL	Foods that are known to have specific disease-fighting qualities for your blood type.
BENEFICIAL	Foods with components that enhance the metabolic, immune, or structural health of you blood type.
NEUTRAL: Allowed Infrequently	Foods that normally have no direct type effect but may impede your progress when consumed regularly.
AVOID	Foods with components that are harmful to your blood type.

Your secretor status can influence your ability to fully digest and metabolize certain foods, so various adjustments in the values are made for non-secretors. If you do not know your secretor type, the odds are that you can safely use the "secretor" values, since the majority of the population (approximately 80 percent) are secretors. However, I urge you to get tested, since the variations are important for non-secretors who want to maximize the effectiveness of the Blood Type Diet.

The food charts are divided into three sections. The top of the chart suggests the average portion size and quantity per week or day, according to secretor status. These recommendations do *not* apply to the category **Neutral: Allowed Infrequently;** those foods should be eaten rarely, if at all. The charts also indicate differences in frequency for some foods, based on ethnic heritage. It has been my experience that this factor has an impact upon the individual's ability to fully digest certain foods. For the purposes of blood type food choices, persons of Hispanic heritage should follow the recommendations for Caucasians, and North American Native peoples should follow the recommendations for Asians.

The middle section of the chart gives the food values. The bottom section lists variants based on secretor status.

For your convenience, we have included a number of product names (Ezekiel bread, Worcestershire sauce, etc.). However, keep in mind that commercial formulations vary among brands and regions. Even though a product may be listed as acceptable for you, always check its ingredients; do not use products that contain **Avoid** ingredients for your blood type. Of course, you may choose to make your own version of commercial products, such as bread and mayonnaise, using ingredients that suit your blood type. There are hundreds of delicious recipes for every blood type available on our Web site (www.dadamo. com) and in the book *Cook Right 4 Your Type: The Practical Kitchen Companion to* Eat Right 4 Your Type.

Meat/Poultry

Blood Type AB is somewhat better adapted to animal-based proteins than Blood Type A, mainly because of the B gene's effects on the production of enzymes involved in fat transport and digestion. However, you need to limit meat. Consider it more of a side dish or garnish than a main course. Like Blood Type B, you must avoid chicken, which contains a B-immunoreactive lectin. Choose only the best-quality (preferably free-range) chemical-, antibiotic-, and pesticide-free, low-fat meats and poultry.

BLOOD TYPE AB: MEAT/POULTRY			
Portion: 4–6 oz (men); 2–5 oz (women and children)			
	African	Caucasian	Asian
Secretor	2–5	1–5	1–5
Non-Secretor	3–5	2–5	2–5
		Times per week	

SUPER BENEFICIAL	BENEFICIAL	NEUTRAL: Allowed Frequently	NEUTRAL: Allowed Infrequently	AVOID
	Lamb Mutton Rabbit Turkey	Goat Liver (calf) Ostrich Pheasant		All commercially processed meats Bacon/Ham/Pork Beef Buffalo Chicken Cornish hen Duck Goose Grouse Guinea hen Heart (beef) Partridge Quail Squab Squirrel Sweetbreads Turtle Veal Venison

Special Variants: *Non-Secretor* NEUTRAL (Allowed Frequently): quail, venison.

Fish/Seafood

Fish and seafood provide an excellent means of optimizing NK cell activity. Richly oiled cold-water fish, such as mackerel, salmon, and sardines, are good sources of omega-3 fatty acids. In general, many of the seafoods that Blood Type AB must avoid have lectins with either A- or B- specificity or polyamines commonly found in the foods. Avoid consuming flash-frozen fish, which has high polyamine content.

BLOOD TYPE AB: FISH/SEAFOOD			
Portion: 4–6 oz (men); 2–5 oz (women and children)			
	African	Caucasian	Asian
Secretor	4–6	3–5	3–5
Non-Secretor	4–7	4–6	4–6
		Times per week	

SUPER BENEFICIAL	BENEFICIAL	NEUTRAL: Allowed Frequently	NEUTRAL: Allowed Infrequently	AVOID
Mackerel	Cod	Abalone		Anchovy
Salmon	Grouper	Bluefish		Barracuda
Sardine	Mahi-mahi	Bullhead		Bass (all)
	Monkfish	Butterfish		Beluga
	Pickerel	Carp		Clam
	Pike	Catfish		Conch
	Porgy	Caviar (stur-		Crab
	Red snap-	geon)		Eel
	per	Chub		Flounder
	Sailfish	Croaker		Frog
	Shad	Cusk		Gray sole
	Snail (*Helix*	Drum		Haddock
	pomatia/	Halfmoon		Hake
	escargot)	fish		Halibut
	Sturgeon	Harvest fish		Herring
	Tuna	Herring		(pickled/
		(fresh)		smoked)
		Mullet		Lobster
		Muskel-		Octopus
		lunge		Oysters

SUPER BENEFICIAL	BENEFICIAL	NEUTRAL: Allowed Frequently	NEUTRAL: Allowed Infrequently	AVOID
		Mussels		Salmon (smoked)
		Opaleye fish		Salmon roe
		Orange roughy		Shrimp
		Parrot fish		Sole
		Perch (all)		Trout (all)
		Pollock		Whiting
		Pompano		Yellowtail
		Rosefish		
		Scallops		
		Scrod		
		Scup		
		Shark		
		Smelt		
		Snapper		
		Squid (calamari)		
		Sucker		
		Sunfish		
		Swordfish		
		Tilapia		
		Tilefish		
		Weakfish		
		Whitefish		

Special Variants: *Non-Secretor* BENEFICIAL: herring (fresh); NEUTRAL (Allowed Frequently): trout (all).

Dairy/Eggs

Dairy products can be used with discretion by many Blood Type AB individuals, especially secretors. Some cultured dairy foods are especially BENEFICIAL, such as kefir and yogurt. Ghee (clarified butter) is an antioxidant, rich in omega-3 oils and short-chain fatty acids. Eggs, which, like fish, are a good source of docosahexaenoic acid (DHA), can complement the protein profile for your blood type. Do your best to find eggs and dairy foods that meet organic standards.

BLOOD TYPE AB: EGGS			
Portion: 1 egg			
	African	Caucasian	Asian
Secretor	2–5	3–4	3–4
Non-Secretor	3–6	3–6	3–6
		Times per week	

BLOOD TYPE AB: MILK AND YOGURT			
Portion: 4–6 oz (men); 2–5 oz (women and children)			
	African	Caucasian	Asian
Secretor	2–6	3–6	1–6
Non-Secretor	0–3	0–4	0–3
		Times per week	

BLOOD TYPE AB: CHEESE			
Portion: 3 oz (men); 2 oz (women and children)			
	African	Caucasian	Asian
Secretor	2–3	3–4	3–4
Non-Secretor	0	0–1	0
		Times per week	

SUPER BENEFICIAL	BENEFICIAL	NEUTRAL: Allowed Frequently	NEUTRAL: Allowed Infrequently	AVOID
Ghee (clarified butter)	Cottage cheese	Casein	Cheddar	American cheese
Kefir	Egg (chicken)	Cream cheese	Colby	Blue cheese
Yogurt	Farmer cheese	Edam	Emmenthal	Brie
	Feta	Egg (goose/quail)	Milk (cow)	Butter
	Goat cheese	Gouda	Monterey Jack	Buttermilk
	Milk (goat)	Gruyère	Quark	Camembert
	Mozzarella	Jarlsberg	Sherbet	Egg (duck)
		Muenster	String cheese	Half-and-half
				Ice cream

SUPER BENEFICIAL	BENEFICIAL	NEUTRAL: Allowed Frequently	NEUTRAL: Allowed Infrequently	AVOID
	Ricotta Sour cream	Neufchâtel Paneer Quark	Swiss cheese	Parmesan Provolone

Special Variants: *Non-Secretor* NEUTRAL (Allowed Frequently): goat cheese, yogurt; AVOID: Emmenthal, Swiss cheese.

Oils

Olive oil, a monounsaturated fat, is SUPER BENEFICIAL for Blood Type AB. Constituents in olive oil, such as flavonoids, squalenes, and polyphenols, act as powerful antioxidants. Use it as your primary cooking oil. Also SUPER BENEFICIAL is flax (linseed) oil, which is high in alpha-linolenic acid (ALA) and has anti-inflammatory properties.

Make it a point to avoid corn, sesame, and safflower oils, which can contain immunoreactive proteins that impair Blood Type AB digestion. These oils can interfere with proper immune function and stimulate the inflammatory response.

BLOOD TYPE AB: OILS			
Portion: 1 tblsp			
	African	Caucasian	Asian
Secretor	4–7	5–8	5–7
Non-Secretor	3–6	3–6	3–4
	Times per week		

SUPER BENEFICIAL	BENEFICIAL	NEUTRAL: Allowed Frequently	NEUTRAL: Allowed Infrequently	AVOID
Flax (linseed) Olive	Walnut	Almond Black currant seed Borage seed Canola Castor Cod liver Evening primrose Peanut Soy	Wheat germ	Avocado Coconut Corn Cottonseed Safflower Sesame Sunflower

Special Variants: None.

Nuts and Seeds

Nuts and seeds can be an important secondary source of protein for Blood Type AB. Laboratory research has identified at least five natural phytochemicals in nuts that regulate the immune system and act as antioxidants. SUPER BENEFICIAL for Blood Type AB are flaxseeds and walnuts, which are high in omega-3 fatty acids. Flaxseeds are particularly rich in lignins, which can help lower the number of receptors for epidermal growth factor, which can trigger inflammatory conditions.

BLOOD TYPE AB: NUTS AND SEEDS			
Portion: Whole (handful); Nut Butters (2 tblsp)			
	African	Caucasian	Asian
Secretor	5–10	5–10	5–9
Non-Secretor	4–8	4–9	5–9
		Times per week	

SUPER BENEFICIAL	BENEFICIAL	NEUTRAL: Allowed Frequently	NEUTRAL: Allowed Infrequently	AVOID
Flax (linseed) Walnut (black/ English)	Chestnut Peanut Peanut butter	Almond Almond butter Almond cheese Almond milk Beechnut Butternut Hickory Litchi Pignolia (pine nut)	Brazil nut Cashew Cashew butter Macadamia Pecan Pecan butter Pistachio Safflower seed	Filbert (hazelnut) Poppy seed Pumpkin seed Sesame butter (tahini) Sesame seed Sunflower butter Sunflower seed

Special Variants: *Non-Secretor* NEUTRAL (Allowed Frequently): peanut; AVOID: Brazil nut, cashew, cashew butter, pistachio.

Beans and Legumes

Blood Type AB does well on proteins found in many beans and legumes, although this food category contains more than a few beans with problematic A- or B- specific lectins. In general, soy beans and their related products are SUPER BENEFICIAL for the Blood Type AB immune system.

BLOOD TYPE AB: BEANS AND LEGUMES			
Portion: 1 cup (cooked)			
	African	Caucasian	Asian
Secretor	3–6	3–6	4–6
Non-Secretor	2–5	2–5	3–6
		Times per week	

SUPER BENEFICIAL	BENEFICIAL	NEUTRAL: Allowed Frequently	NEUTRAL: Allowed Infrequently	AVOID
Miso Soy bean Soy cheese Soy milk Tempeh Tofu	Lentil (green) Navy bean Pinto bean	Bean (green/ snap/ string) Cannellini bean Copper bean Lentil (domestic/ red) Northern bean Pea (green/ pod/ snow) Tamarind bean White bean	Jicama bean	Adzuki bean Black bean Black-eyed pea Fava (broad) bean Garbanzo (chickpea) Kidney bean Lima bean Mung bean/ sprout

Special Variants: *Non-Secretor* NEUTRAL (Allowed Frequently): fava (broad) bean, navy bean; AVOID: jicama bean.

Grains and Starches

Blood Type AB individuals benefit from a moderate consumption of the proper grains for their type. Non-secretors should limit wheat—and all individuals with arthritis should avoid whole wheat. Blood Type AB is also sensitive to the lectin in corn and should avoid all corn flour products. Essene (manna) bread, a heavy, dense, fully sprouted bread, is laced with a free radical scavenging enzyme called super oxide dismutase (SOD).

BLOOD TYPE AB: GRAINS AND STARCHES			
Portion: ½ cup dry (grains or pastas); 1 muffin; 2 slices of bread			
	African	Caucasian	Asian
Secretor	6–8	6–9	6–10
Non-Secretor	4–6	5–7	6–8
		Times per week	

SUPER BENEFICIAL	BENEFICIAL	NEUTRAL: Allowed Frequently	NEUTRAL: Allowed Infrequently	AVOID
Essene bread (manna)	Amaranth Ezekiel bread Millet Oat bran Oat flour Oatmeal Rice (whole) Rice (wild) Rice bran Rice cake Rye (whole) Rye flour Soy flour/ products Spelt (whole) Spelt flour/ products	Barley Quinoa 100% sprouted grain products	Couscous Wheat (re-fined/un-bleached) Wheat (semolina) Wheat (white flour) Wheat (whole) Wheat bran Wheat germ	Buckwheat Cornmeal Grits Kamut Popcorn Soba noodles (100% buck-wheat) Sorghum Tapioca Teff

Special Variants: *Non-Secretor* NEUTRAL (Allowed Frequently): Ezekiel bread, spelt (whole), spelt flour/products; AVOID: soy flour/products, wheat (refined/un-bleached), wheat (white flour), wheat (whole), wheat germ.

Vegetables

Vegetables can be your first line of defense against chronic disease. They provide a rich source of antioxidants and fiber and are essential to intestinal health. Blood Type AB SUPER BENEFICIALS include onions and garlic, which are high in quercetin, a flavonoid with potent anti-inflammatory properties, and other antioxidants that decrease oxidative stress and increase glutathione, which protects cells. Onions and garlic are also rich sources of diallyl sulfide, which detoxifies carcinogens. Broccoli contains allyl methyl trisulfide and dithiolthiones, which increase the activity of enzymes involved in detoxification of carcinogens. Sweet potatoes are rich in vitamins A and B_6, which stabilize immune function. Cabbage and cauliflower positively influence Blood Type AB's disease susceptibility. Mushrooms (maitake and the common domestic variety, called silver dollar) are powerful infection fighters. Tomatoes, a rich source of lycopene, are SUPER BENEFICIAL for Blood Type AB, although they are not recommended for Blood Types A and B.

An item's value also applies to its juice, unless otherwise noted.

BLOOD TYPE B: VEGETABLES			
Portion: 1 cup, prepared (cooked or raw)			
	African	Caucasian	Asian
Secretor Super/ Beneficials	Unlimited	Unlimited	Unlimited
Secretor Neutrals	2–5	2–5	2–5
Non-Secretor Super/ Beneficials	Unlimited	Unlimited	Unlimited
Non-Secretor Neutrals	2–3	2–3	2–3
	Times per day		

SUPER BENEFICIAL	BENEFICIAL	NEUTRAL: Allowed Frequently	NEUTRAL: Allowed Infrequently	AVOID
Broccoli	Alfalfa	Arugula	Carrot	Aloe
Cabbage	sprouts	Asparagus	Daikon	Artichoke
Cabbage	Beet	Asparagus	radish	Corn
(juice)*	Beet	pea	Olive	Mushroom
Cauliflower	greens	Bamboo	(Greek/	(abalone/
Garlic	Carrot	shoot	green/	shiitake)
Mushroom	(juice)	Bok choy	Spanish)	Olive
(maitake,	Celery	Brussels	Poi	(black)
silver dol-	Collards	sprouts	Potato	Peppers (all)
lar)	Cucumber	Celeriac	Pumpkin	Pickles (all)
Onion (all)	Dandelion	Chicory	Taro	Radish/
Tomato	Eggplant	Cucumber		sprouts
	Kale	(juice)		Rhubarb
	Mustard	Endive		
	greens	Escarole		
	Parsnip	Fennel		
	Potato	Fiddlehead		
	(sweet)	fern		
	Yam	Horseradish		
		Kohlrabi		
		Leek		
		Lettuce (all)		
		Mushroom		
		(enoki/		
		oyster/		
		porto-		
		bello/		
		straw/tree		
		ear)		
		Okra		
		Oyster plant		
		Radicchio		
		Rappini		
		(broccoli		
		rabe)		
		Rutabaga		
		Scallion		
		Seaweeds		
		Shallot		
		Spinach		

SUPER BENEFICIAL	BENEFICIAL	NEUTRAL: Allowed Frequently	NEUTRAL: Allowed Infrequently	AVOID
		Squash (all) Swiss chard Tomato Turnip Water chestnut Watercress Yucca Zucchini		

Special Variants: *Non-Secretor* BENEFICIAL: tomato, NEUTRAL (Allowed Frequently): beet, onion (all); AVOID: poi, taro.

*To obtain the benefits of cabbage juice, it must be consumed within one minute of juicing.

Fruits and Fruit Juices

Fruits are rich in antioxidants. Many, such as blueberries, elderberries, and cherries, contain pigments that inhibit intestinal toxins. Many fruits, such as pineapple, are rich in enzymes that can help reduce inflammation and encourage proper water balance. Grapes and grape juice are powerful antioxidants.

An item's value also applies to its juice, unless otherwise noted.

BLOOD TYPE AB: FRUITS AND FRUIT JUICES			
Portion: 1 cup			
	African	**Caucasian**	**Asian**
Secretor	3–4	3–6	3–5
Non-Secretor	1–3	2–3	3–4
	Times per day		

SUPER BENEFICIAL	BENEFICIAL	NEUTRAL: Allowed Frequently	NEUTRAL: Allowed Infrequently	AVOID
Blueberry Cherry Elderberry (dark blue/ purple) Grape (all) Pineapple	Cranberry Fig (fresh/ dried) Gooseberry Grapefruit Kiwi Lemon Loganberry Plum Watermelon	Apple Blackberry Boysen- berry Grapefruit (juice) Kumquat Lime Mulberry Muskmelon Nectarine Papaya Peach Pear Persian melon Pineapple (juice) Plantain Raspberry Spanish melon Strawberry Youngberry	Apricot Asian pear Breadfruit Canang melon Cantaloupe Casaba melon Christmas melon Crenshaw melon Currant Date Honeydew Prune Raisin Tangerine	Avocado Banana Bitter melon Coconut Dewberry Guava Loganberry Mango Orange Persimmon Pome- granate Prickly pear Quince Sago palm Star fruit (carambola)

Special Variants: *Non-Secretor* BENEFICIAL: blackberry, lime; NEUTRAL (Allowed Frequently): banana; AVOID: cantaloupe, honeydew, prune, tangerine.

Spices/Condiments/Sweeteners

Many spices are known to have anti-inflammatory properties. The common cooking spices—rosemary, thyme, and oregano—are powerful antioxidants that exert anti-inflammatory effects. Turmeric and garlic are also anti-inflammatory. Ginger inhibits the production of COX-2, an enzyme that triggers the inflammatory response. Parsley contains quercetin, which is anti-inflammatory. Licorice root provides antiviral support.

Many common food additives, such as guar gum and carrageenan, enhance the effects of lectins found in other foods and should be avoided. Use caution when using prepared condiments. They often contain wheat, which is a primary factor in the development of arthritis and other inflammatory conditions.

SUPER BENEFICIAL	BENEFICIAL	NEUTRAL: Allowed Frequently	NEUTRAL: Allowed Infrequently	AVOID
Garlic	Dill	Basil	Agar	Allspice
Ginger	Horse-	Bay leaf	Apple	Almond
Parsley	radish	Bergamot	pectin	extract
Turmeric	Molasses	Caraway	Arrowroot	Anise
	(black-	Cardamom	Chocolate	Aspartame
	strap)	Carob	Honey	Barley malt
	Oregano	Chervil	Maple	Caper
	Tarragon	Chili	syrup	Carrageenan
		powder	Mayonnaise	Cornstarch
		Chive	Molasses	Corn syrup
		Cilantro	Rice syrup	Dextrose
		(coriander	Soy sauce	Fructose
		leaf)	Sugar	Gelatin (ex-
		Cinnamon	(brown/	cept veg-
		Clove	white)	sourced)
		Coriander	Yeast	Guarana
		Cream of	(baker's/	Gums
		tartar	brewer's)	(acacia/
		Cumin		Arabic/
		Juniper		guar)
		Lecithin		Invert sugar
		Licorice		Ketchup
		root*		Malto-
		Mace		dextrin
		Marjoram		MSG
		Mint (all)		Pepper
		Mustard		(black/
		(dry)		white)
		Nutmeg		Pepper
		Paprika		(cayenne)

SUPER BENEFICIAL	BENEFICIAL	NEUTRAL: Allowed Frequently	NEUTRAL: Allowed Infrequently	AVOID

		Rosemary
		Saffron
		Sage
		Savory
		Sea salt
		Seaweeds
		Senna
		Stevia
		Tamari
		  (wheat-
		  free)
		Tamarind
		Thyme
		Vanilla
		Vegetable
		  glycerine
		Winter-
		  green
				Pepper (pep-
				  percorn/
				  red flakes)
				Pickles (all)
				Sucanat
				Tapioca
				Vinegar (all)
				Worcester-
				  shire
				  sauce

Special Variants: *Non-Secretor* BENEFICIAL: bay leaf, yeast (brewer's); NEUTRAL (Allowed Frequently): dill, tarragon; AVOID: agar, honey, juniper, maple syrup, rice syrup, sugar (brown/white).

*Do not use if you have high blood pressure.

Herbal Teas

Several herbal teas can be SUPER BENEFICIAL arthritis fighters for Blood Type AB. Ginger contains pungent phenolic substances with pronounced antioxidant and anti-inflammatory activities. Echinacea helps fight infection, and licorice root provides a strong defense against viral infections.

SUPER BENEFICIAL	BENEFICIAL	NEUTRAL: Allowed Frequently	NEUTRAL: Allowed Infrequently	AVOID
Echinacea Ginger Licorice root*	Alfalfa Burdock Chamomile Ginseng Hawthorn Parsley Rosehip Strawberry leaf	Catnip Chickweed Dandelion Dong quai Elder Fenugreek Goldenseal Horehound Mulberry Peppermint Raspberry leaf Sage Sarsaparilla Senna Slippery elm Spearmint St. John's wort Thyme Valerian Vervain White birch White oak bark Yarrow Yellow dock		Aloe Coltsfoot Corn silk Gentian Hops Linden Mullein Red clover Rhubarb Shepherd's purse Skullcap

Special Variants: None

*Do not use if you have high blood pressure.

Miscellaneous Beverages

Green tea is a SUPER BENEFICIAL beverage for Blood Type AB, because of its antioxidant properties. It also inhibits TNF-alpha gene expression. TNF-alpha is known to be a central mediator in chronic inflammatory diseases such as rheumatoid arthritis and multiple sclerosis. Drink green tea as a daily substitute for coffee. Avoid or limit alcohol to red wine. Alcohol can exacerbate autoimmune inflammatory conditions and may be a factor in the development of some forms of arthritis, such as gout.

SUPER BENEFICIAL	BENEFICIAL	NEUTRAL: Allowed Frequently	NEUTRAL: Allowed Infrequently	AVOID
Tea (green)	Wine (red)	Beer Seltzer Soda (club) Wine (white)		Coffee (reg/decaf) Liquor Soda (cola/ diet/misc.) Tea, black (reg/decaf)
Special Variants: *Non-Secretor* AVOID: beer.				

Supplements

THE BLOOD TYPE AB Diet offers abundant quantities of important nutrients, such as protein and iron. It is important to get as many nutrients as possible from fresh foods and use supplements only to fill in the minor deficiencies in your diet. The following supplement protocols are designed for Blood Type AB individuals who are suffering from arthritis or related autoimmune conditions.

Note: If you are being treated for a medical condition, consult your doctor before taking any supplements.

Blood Type AB: Anti-Inflammatory Protocol

Use this protocol for 12 weeks to prevent and minimize inflammatory conditions, while balancing immune function.

SUPPLEMENT	ACTION	DOSAGE
MSM (*methylsulfony-methane*)	Promotes joint and pulmonary health	500 mg, twice daily
Niacin (vitamin B$_3$)*	Promotes healthy digestion and metabolism	50 mg, 2 capsules daily
Larch arabinogalactan (*Larix officinalis*)	Promotes digestive and intestinal health	1 tablespoon, twice daily, in juice or water
Quercetin	Has anti-inflammatory effects	500 mg, twice daily, away from food
Frankincense (*Boswellia serrata*)	Has anti-inflammatory effects	500 mg, 1–2 capsules, away from food
Jiaogulan (*Gynostemma pentaphyllum*)	Acts as an anti-inflammatory	60 mg gynostemma whole glucosides, twice daily
Ginger root (*Rhizome zingiberis*)	COX-2 inhibitor and pain reliever	200 mg standarized extract capsules, before meals, or as a tea, fresh juice, or compress

*Do not exceed recommended dosage.

Blood Type AB: Arthritis Pain Relief Adjunct

Use this protocol for 4 weeks to reduce pain associated with joint disease.

SUPPLEMENT	ACTION	DOSAGE
Ginger root (*Rhizome zingiberis*)	COX-2 inhibitor; pain reliever	200 mg standardized extract capsules before meals, or as a tea, fresh juice, or compress
Bromelain (pineapple enzyme)	Has antioxidant and anti-inflammatory properties	500 mg, 1–3 capsules daily with meals, gradually decreasing dose and frequency as symptoms improve

Blood Type AB: Joint Repair Adjunct

Use this protocol for 4 weeks to promote healing and improve joint integrity.

SUPPLEMENT	ACTION	DOSAGE
Chondroitin sulfate	Supports regeneration of joint cartilage	600 mg, 2 capsules daily, away from food
Glucosamine sulfate	Enables joint repair	500 mg, 2–3 capsules daily, away from food
Vitamin C (rose hips or acerola cherry)	Powerful antioxidant; promotes healing	250 mg, twice daily

Blood Type AB: Surgery Recovery Adjunct

When surgery is scheduled, add this protocol for 2 weeks before surgery and 2 weeks after.		
SUPPLEMENT	**ACTION**	**DOSAGE**
Gotu kola (*Centella asiatica*)*	Aids wound healing and proper blood flow	100 mg, twice daily
Chamomile (*Matricaria chamomilla*)	A mild digestive and antidepressant	Herbal tincture:25 drops in warm water, 2–3 times daily
Horsetail (*Equisetum arvense*)	Promotes healing; facilitates calcium absorption	500 mg, twice daily

*Do not use if you are pregnant.

The Exercise Component

THE BEST WISDOM of both conventional and naturopathic medicine is that regular exercise, including aerobic activity and weights, is essential to fighting arthritis and autoimmune diseases. It may seem counterintuitive, since arthritis makes movement difficult and often painful. However, studies consistently show that aerobic exercise can reduce joint swelling. Strength training builds muscle, helping to support and protect joints affected by arthritis. Physical exercise also promotes lean muscle mass and reduces weight, thus lightening the load on stressed joints.

For Blood Type AB, overall fitness is achieved with a balance of moderate aerobic activity and mentally soothing, stress-reducing exercises. Below is a list of exercises for Blood Type AB.

3 Steps to Effective Exercise:

1. Warm up with stretching and flexibility movements before you start your aerobic exercise.

EXERCISE	DURATION	FREQUENCY
Martial arts	30–60 minutes	2–3 x week
Cycling	45–60 minutes	2–3 x week
Hiking	30–60 minutes	2–3 x week
Golf (no cart!)	60–90 minutes	2–3 x week
Walking	40–50 minutes	2–3 x week
Pilates	40–50 minutes	2–3 x week
Swimming	45 minutes	2–3 x week
Yoga	40–50 minutes	1–2 x week
T'ai Chi	40–50 minutes	1–2 x week

2. To achieve maximum cardiovascular benefits, work toward an elevated heart rate that is about 70 percent of your capacity. Once you reach the elevated rate, continue exercising to maintain that rate for twenty to thirty minutes. To calculate your maximum heart rate and performance level:
   - Subtract your age from 220.
   - Multiply the difference by .70 (or .60 if you are over age sixty). This is the high end of your performance.
   - Multiply the remainder by .50. This is the low end of your performance.
3. Finish each aerobic session with at least a five-minute cooldown of stretching and relaxation moves.

Getting Started: The First Month

IF YOU ARE NEW to the Blood Type Diet, the following guidelines will introduce you to the Blood Type AB regimen over a period of one month. Follow these recommendations as closely as possible, using a journal to record your personal experiences with the diet. In addition to factors that are measurable in laboratory tests, take the time to note changes in your energy levels, pain levels, sleep patterns, digestion, and overall well-being.

Blood Type AB Arthritis Diet Checklist

Derive your protein primarily from sources other than red ☐
meat. Low levels of hydrochloric acid and intestinal alkaline
phosphatase make it difficult for Blood Type AB to digest meats.

Eat soy foods and seafood as your primary protein. ☐

Include regular portions of richly oiled cold-water fish every ☐
week.

Include modest amounts of cultured dairy foods in your diet, ☐
but limit fresh milk products, which cause excess mucus
production and can trigger inflammation.

Don't overdo the grains, especially wheat-derived foods. ☐

Avoid wheat if you have arthritis. ☐

Eat lots of BENEFICIAL fruits and vegetables, especially those ☐
high in antioxidants and fiber.

Avoid coffee. Substitute green tea every day for extra immune ☐
system benefits.

Week 1

Blood Type Diet and Supplements

- Eliminate your most harmful AVOID foods—chicken, corn, buckwheat, most
  shellfish, and lectin-activated beans.
- Avoid wheat if you have arthritis.
- Include your most important BENEFICIAL foods frequently throughout the
  week. For example, have soy-based foods 5 times and omega-3-rich fish
  3 to 4 times, with lots of BENEFICIAL vegetables and fruit.
- Incorporate at least 1 SUPER BENEFICIAL food into your daily diet. For example,
  eat slices of fresh pineapple over yogurt, or sprinkle walnuts on a salad.
- If you're a coffee drinker, begin to wean yourself by cutting your daily
  consumption in half. Substitute green tea or one of the SUPER BENEFICIAL
  herbal teas.

Exercise Regimen

- Plan to exercise at least 4 days this week, for 45 minutes each day.

  2 days: walking or light aerobic activity

  2 days: yoga or T'ai Chi

- If you have joint impairment, start slowly, and gradually increase your duration and intensity of activity. The important factor is consistency. Just do it—as much as you're able.

- Use your journal to detail the time, activity, distance, and amount of weight. Note the number of repetitions for each exercise.

▪ WEEK 1 SUCCESS STRATEGY ▪
Spice up your juicing

Juice about a one-inch piece of fresh ginger and add it to your favorite SUPER BENEFICIAL or BENEFICIAL juice. Blend to make a smoothie. Or just add the ginger to hot water as tea. Ginger provides a cornucopia of natural anti-inflammatory compounds, adds pungency to many food dishes, and freshly juiced ginger makes the kitchen smell wonderful!

Week 2

Blood Type Diet and Supplements

- Begin to eliminate the next level of AVOID foods—grains, vegetables, and fruits that react poorly with Type AB blood.

- Eat 2 to 3 BENEFICIAL proteins every day.

- Continue to incorporate SUPER BENEFICIAL foods into your daily diet.

- Choose the NEUTRAL foods listed as Allowed Frequently, over those listed as Allowed Infrequently.

- If you're a coffee drinker, continue to cut your coffee intake, replacing it with BENEFICIAL herbal teas. Drink a cup of green tea every morning.

- Manage your mealtimes to aid proper digestion. Avoid eating on the run. Make your meals relaxing, sit-down affairs. Eat slowly and chew thoroughly to encourage digestive secretions.

Exercise Regimen

- Continue to exercise at least 4 days this week, for 45 minutes each day.

  2 days: walking or light aerobic activity

  2 days: yoga or T'ai Chi

- If your work is sedentary, get in the habit of taking a couple of "movement" breaks during the day. Walk around the block or up and down stairs. Movement will help maintain joint flexibility.

> **■ WEEK 2 SUCCESS STRATEGY ■**
> **Arnicate your joints**
>
> Arnica (*Arnica montana*), also commonly called "Leopard's bane," is an herb that has been used in homeopathic medicine for hundreds of years. Arnica appears to stimulate blood circulation and have anti-inflammatory qualities that may reduce arthritis pain and swelling. Arnica can be taken as a gel or ointment applied externally on the skin. I find that the joint creams work great for Blood Type AB when applied before bedtime. Avoid taking arnica internally.

Week 3

Blood Type Diet and Supplements

- When you plan your meals for week 3, choose BENEFICIAL foods to replace NEUTRAL foods whenever possible.
- Eliminate all remaining AVOID foods.
- Liberally incorporate SUPER BENEFICIAL foods into your daily diet.
- Completely wean yourself from coffee, substituting green or herbal tea.

Exercise Regimen

- Continue to exercise at least 4 days this week, for 45 minutes each day.

  2 days: walking or light aerobic activity

  2 days: yoga or T'ai Chi

■ **WEEK 3 SUCCESS STRATEGY** ■
Balance your natural born killers

Natural killer cells are white blood cells of the immune system. They are different from T- and B-lymphocytes because they do not have unique receptors for a particular antigenic target. Thus, these cells provide a non-specific immune response to various pathogens and require certain cytokines to become activated and to increase in numbers. They participate in several of the immune responses and can help antibodies kill target cells.

Blood Type AB tends to have higher than average levels of NK cell activity, probably the result of the body's compensation for a lack of antibodies to opposing blood types. Overactive NK activity can increase the chances of inflammation and autoimmune disease, so a proper balance of NK cell activity is crucial for Blood Type AB.

Maintaining healthy and balanced NK cell activity reads like a basic primer of naturopathic medicine

1. Adequate fresh air and sunlight
2. Exercise
3. Low sugar diet
4. Stress modulation
5. Avoidance of stimulants, such as excess caffeine, nicotine, etc.

It may seem that keeping your NK cells happy is a lot of work, but you'll see the dividends in the form of less pain, greater mobility, and a better sense of well-being.

Week 4

Blood Type Diet and Supplements

- Continue at the week 3 level, focusing on BENEFICIAL and SUPER BENEFICIAL foods.

Exercise Regimen

- Continue at the week 3 level.
- Review your progress, noting in your journal improvements in strength and flexibility. Determine which exercise regimen has worked for you, including time of day, setting, and activity level.

▪ WEEK 4 SUCCESS STRATEGY ▪
Build Strong Bones

Type AB women have an increased risk of bone loss as they age because of low levels of intestinal alkaline phosphatase. Repeated studies have shown that this enzyme positively impacts calcium metabolism. Furthermore, higher stomach acid predicts better calcium absorption. Although conventional wisdom in the nutrition community holds that high-protein diets accelerate bone loss, the scientific literature shows that the opposite is true. This presents a special challenge for Type AB women. To promote healthy bones:

1. Eat canned salmon and sardines with the bones.
2. Regularly consume low-fat yogurt, soy milk, and goat milk.
3. Include lots of broccoli and spinach in your diet.
4. Take daily dose of supplemental calcium citrate—300 to 600 mg.
5. Follow the Type AB exercise regimen, and do as much walking as you can.

A Final Word

IN SUMMARY, the secret to fighting arthritis with the Blood Type AB Diet involves:

1. Increasing overall health and fitness by eating a diet rich in soy protein, BENEFICIAL seafood, cultured dairy, and green vegetables.
2. Minimizing the consumption of pro-inflammatory lectins, most abundant in grains such as wheat, buckwheat, and corn.
3. Increasing circulatory efficiency, lowering cholesterol and blood pressure, and reducing stress by adopting an exercise regimen that combines calming activities with vigorous routines.
4. Using supplements to block the effects of pro-inflammatory lectins, provide antioxidant support, and help repair damaged tissue.

Appendices

A Simple Definition of Terms

agglutination: Clumping, or "gluing," together. One means by which the immune system defends against foreign matter and toxins, notably against lectins and opposing blood type material.

ankylosing spondylitis: A chronic inflammatory type of arthritis that mainly affects the spine.

antibody: The product of the immune system when it is stimulated by specific antigens. There are many classes of antibodies, among them "agglutinins," which isolate foreign substances by clumping them together so that they may be eliminated. Blood Types O, A, and B manufacture antibodies to other blood types. Blood Type AB, the universal recipient, manufactures no antibodies to other blood types.

antigen: A chemical that provokes an immune system antibody response. The blood type "I.D." present on the blood cells, identified as Type A or B, is one example. A Type AB cell has both of these antigens. The blood type having no antigen is described as O—or "zero." As we age, it is to our advantage to shore up our store of circulating anti–blood type antigens, as lower levels mean increased susceptibility to diseases arising from substances and organisms bearing opposing antigens.

antioxidant: A substance known to moderate the oxidation, or aging, process in human cells by lowering free radical levels. Vitamins C and E, and many plants and plant-derived substances such as green tea, quercetin, arabinogalactan, and milk thistle, are potent antioxidants.

autoimmune diseases: Diseases generated when the cells that normally defend the body against infections mistakenly attack their own cells, tissues, and organs.

blood type: The term commonly used to refer to the ABO blood group system. Originally used primarily to determine suitable blood and organ donor–recipient matches, ABO type determines many of the digestive and immunological characteristics of the body, as well as susceptibility to the diseases arising from infection, immune suppression, and digestive impairment. It is also one of the tools of anthropology in establishing the origins, socioeconomic development, and movements of ancient peoples.

bursitis: Inflammation of the bursae—small, fluid-filled sacs that help reduce friction between bones and other moving structures in the joints.

complement: Proteins involved in the inflammatory response.

COX-2: An enzyme in the blood that triggers inflammation.

cytokines: Messenger proteins that induce the release of acute phase proteins, such as complement, and act as fever producers.

fibromyalgia: A chronic condition that causes widespread pain and fatigue. The term *fibromyalgia* comes from "fibro" (fibrous tissues, such as tendons and ligaments), "my" (muscles), and "algia" (pain). Unlike arthritis, fibromyalgia does not cause pain or swelling in the joints themselves; rather, it produces pain in the soft tissues located around joints, skin, and organs throughout the body.

gout: A form of arthritis that occurs when crystals of uric acid accumulate in a joint, leading to the sudden development of pain and inflammation. Individuals with gout either overproduce uric acid or are less efficient at eliminating it.

hyaluronic acid: Part of cartilage (the "cushion" at the end of the bones where they come together to form a joint) and synovial fluid (the fluid secreted by the lining of the joint to nourish and lubricate the joint). In cartilage, hyaluronan binds to other molecules, helping the cartilage to withstand the force of weight bearing and movement of the joint. In the synovial fluid, hyaluronan lubricates the movement of the cartilage against the lining of the joint (synovium) and also may have some "shock absorber" properties.

immune system: The physiological determination of and response to "self" and "non-self" accomplished through the action of many organs and cells throughout the body, essential to the preservation of its health and integrity.

infectious arthritis: A form of arthritis, called reactive arthritis, that develops as a result of a bacterial or viral infection.

juvenile chronic arthritis: A chronic inflammatory condition in one or more joints that begins before the age of sixteen.

lectins: Proteins that attach to preferred receptors in the human body. Food lectins are often blood type–specific. A lectin's action may initiate agglutination, inflammation, abnormal proliferation of cells of the immune and nervous systems, or insulin resistance, depending upon the type of cells targeted. Abundant in the vegetable kingdom, lectins are fewer in number and type among animal foods, such as eggs, fish, and meats.

non-steroidal anti-inflammatory agents (NSAIDs): Drugs, such as ibuprofen, commonly used to reduce pain and decrease inflammation.

osteoarthritis: A degenerative joint disease in which the surface layer of cartilage breaks down and wears away. This allows bones under the cartilage to rub together, causing pain, swelling, and loss of motion of the joint. Over time, the joint may lose its normal shape.

psoriatic arthritis: An inflammatory arthritis associated with psoriasis, a chronic skin and nail condition.

rheumatoid arthritis: A systemic autoimmune inflammatory condition, attacking the synovium (the membranes surrounding joints).

scleroderma: A chronic autoimmune arthritic disease, also known as systemic sclerosis, involving an overproduction of collagen that causes skin hardening.

selectins: Proteins that mediate the binding of white blood cells to the walls of the blood vessels, signaling the initiation of the inflammatory response.

Sjögren's syndrome: A chronic, systemic inflammatory disorder, characterized by dryness of the mouth, eyes, and other mucous membranes.

synovium: Membranes surrounding the joints.

systemic lupus erythematosus (SLE): An inflammatory autoimmune disease that can involve joints, kidneys, and tissues. Symptoms of lupus include fever, skin rash, anemia, and joint disease.

tendonitis: An inflammation of the tendons—tough cords of tissue that connect muscle to bone. It can be caused by overuse, injury, or arthritis-producing conditions.

FAQs: Arthritis and Blood Type

Blood Type O

I am a Blood Type O with fibromyalgia. I worry that aerobic exercise will make my condition worse. Won't I do better with flexibility exercises, such as yoga?

Studies show that graded aerobic exercise significantly reduces fibromyalgia symptoms. In one controlled clinical trial, reported in the *British Medical Journal*, the improvement with aerobic exercise was better than that seen with relaxation/flexibility training and was enough in some patients that they no longer met criteria for fibromyalgia. Reductions in tender point counts and scores on the fibromyalgia impact questionnaire were also greater in the group that engaged in aerobic exercise.

What supplements would you recommend for a very active, forty-one-year-old Type O male with an injured knee: snapped ACL and torn cartilage?

The anterior cruciate ligament (ACL) of the knee is one of four principal knee ligaments. It seems to be the most important in terms of knee stability and is the most commonly disrupted ligament in the knee. In addition to swelling, this injury is associated with joint instability. In addition to the Blood Type Diet, use the arthritis protocol and joint repair adjunct for the best results.

I have been diagnosed with Sjögren's syndrome. Are there naturopathic remedies I can try?

Sjögren's syndrome is a chronic disorder of unknown cause characterized by a particular form of dry mouth and eyes. This loss of tears and saliva may result in changes in the eyes (called aqueous tear deficiency) and in the mouth with deterioration of the teeth, increased oral infection, difficulty in swallowing, and painful mouth. Sjögren's syndrome may also involve inflammation of the joints (arthritis), muscles (myositis), nerves (neuropathy), thyroid (thyroiditis), kidneys (nephritis), or other areas of the body. Also, patients may have severe fatigue and disruption of their sleep pattern. To support recovery, try the following:

- Fucus (bladderwrack): One approach to dryness is to help break up the thick, sticky secretions. Agents that contain iodides include 10 percent saturated solution of potassium iodide (SSKI). Since one of the main problems with Sjögren's is candida overgrowth, using bladderwrack has the additional benefit of providing low levels of iodine, plus some of the anti-candida properties found in this seaweed.
- Nettle root: Nettle root (*Urtica dioca*) contains a lectin that can down-regulate the immune system, helping to modulate autoimmunity. In addition, nettle root has potent anti-candida properties.
- Probiotic: By consuming beneficial bacteria that is right for your blood type, you can decrease the incidence of oral candida infections and thus mouth discomfort.

I have severe rheumatoid arthritis. I've heard that hydrotherapy can be helpful. What exactly is hydrotherapy?

We use hydrotherapy with great success in our clinic. Its healing and recuperative effects are due to its thermal and mechanical effects. It employs the body's reaction to hot and cold stimuli. From the skin the nerves carry impulses deeper into the body. This is instrumental in lessening pain sensitivity, invigorating blood flow and circulation, increasing the production of stress hormones, and stimulating the immune system. Hydrotherapy works so well because it stimulates the body's own healing forces. During the treatment the patient lies comfortably on a soft table while hot towels are applied over the upper torso. The person is then wrapped in a sheet and covered with several layers of blankets. Once the skin is warmed, cold towels are exchanged for the heated towels. The body, well prepared by the preceding warmth, reacts to this temperature change by greatly increasing the blood flow to the skin and the internal organs of the chest and abdomen. Hydrotherapy researchers have shown that a reflex increase in blood flow occurs in internal organs when the circulation to the overlying skin is stimulated. It is this internal reaction that is responsible for the long-lasting and cumulative effects of a series of hydrotherapy treatments. Research has further shown that the beneficial effects on the immune system last for up to twenty-four hours, making this a very effective therapy for any disorder involving immune function.

Blood Type A

Can acupuncture help relieve osteoarthritis pain?

Acupuncture is one of the oldest, most commonly used medical procedures in the world. Originating in China more than 5,000 years ago, acupuncture has only recently been used in the United States as a beneficial treatment. Although it may seem mysterious and strange, acupuncture is a proven method for pain relief. Currently, one of the main reasons Americans seek acupuncture treatment is to relieve chronic pain, especially from conditions such as arthritis or lower-back disorders.

The perspective from which an acupuncturist views health and sickness hinges on concepts of vital energy, energetic balance, and energetic imbalance. Just as Western medical doctors monitor the blood flowing through blood vessels and the messages traveling via the nervous system, the acupuncturist assesses the flow and distribution of vital energy within its pathways, known as meridians and channels. Increasingly, acupuncture is being used to complement conventional therapies. Many doctors have found that acupuncture lowers the need for conventional pain-killing drugs.

What are the risks and benefits of taking hyaluronic acid to treat osteoporosis?

Hyaluronic acid (HA) is a naturally occurring substance that is present in all connective tissues of the human body. It is in high levels in the skin, ligaments, and joint fluid. It is available in the diet from red meat and various vegetable sources. Hyaluronan (hyaluronic acid) is normally part of cartilage (the "cushion" at the end of the bones where they come together to form a joint) and synovial fluid (the fluid secreted by the lining of the joint to nourish and lubricate the joint). In cartilage, hyaluronan binds to other molecules, helping the cartilage to withstand the force of weight bearing and movement of the joint. In the synovial fluid, hyaluronan lubricates the movement of the cartilage against the lining of the joint (synovium) and also may have some "shock absorber" properties.

Hyaluronic acid is produced by the human body in high levels during the major growth phases of our lives. After we reach maturity, this production decreases, and normal diets do not contain high enough levels to enable the body to replace the HA that is lost during normal metabolism. In osteoarthritis, the concentration of hyaluronan is decreased in the cartilage. The concentration also is reduced in synovial fluid, and the properties of the hyaluronan in osteoarthritic joint fluid are abnormal—they are smaller, less shock-absorbing molecules.

In 1997, two brands of hyaluronan were approved by the FDA as devices to treat osteoarthritis of the knee: Synvisc and Hyalgan. Synvisc is injected into the osteoarthritic knee each week for a total of three consecutive weeks. Hyalgan is injected weekly for a total of five consecutive weeks. At one time it was thought that stomach acid destroyed the hyaluronic acid molecule. More recent research has shown that a large portion of the hyaluronic acid is undisturbed by stomach acid and is available for absorption in the small intestine. This means that you can now supplement this in an oral form instead of its traditional form as an intra-articular injection. Most studies to date have been on the injectable form. Hyaluronan does not cure osteoarthritis or repair damaged cartilage. However, it may improve pain and stiffness temporarily.

Do you have any suggestions for the preparation of flax seeds?

Try my specially formulated Membrane Fluidizer Cocktail:

1 tablespoon flax oil (linseed)
1 tablespoon high-quality lecithin granules
6–8 ounces of fruit juice

Shake well and drink.

There are hundreds of delicious recipes for every blood type available on our Web site (www.dadamo.com) and in the book *Cook Right 4 Your Type: The Practical Kitchen Companion to* Eat Right 4 Your Type.

Can I use a topical glucosamine-chondroitin sulfate cream for arthritis pain relief?

Although a new study suggests that this topical cream may be even more effective than oral supplements for osteoarthritis of the knee, Blood Type A may want to opt for a topical preparation containing the herb arnica instead.

Blood Type B

I'm Type B, and I have been a vegetarian for almost twenty years. How do I make an adjustment to the Blood Type Diet?

Many new subscribers to the diet for Blood Type B have been longtime vegetarians. Here are some guidelines:

1. If you are not used to eating dairy products, introduce them gradually, after you have been on the diet for several weeks. Begin with cultured dairy products, such as yogurt and kefir, which are more easily tolerated than fresh dairy products.

2. The protein in your diet should emphasize a combination of seafood and dairy, with very limited amounts of SUPER BENEFICIAL and BENEFICIAL meat. Until you have adapted to the diet, stay away from some of the meats that are NEUTRAL for Blood Type B, such as beef, veal, liver, and pheasant.

3. Take a digestive enzyme with your main meal until you adapt to eating meat and dairy. Bromelain, an enzyme found in pineapple, is available in supplemental form. In addition, drink ginger, peppermint, or parsley tea once or twice a day. These are all good stomach tonics.

4. Some people are lactose intolerant, and this may be independent of blood type. If you are lactose intolerant, I suggest you try one of the lactose preparations on the market.

Tests conducted by my physician show that I have high levels of C-reactive protein. What can I do to lower these levels?

C-reactive protein (CRP) is an inflammatory marker directly related to arthritis as well as coronary heart disease risk. Studies have shown a strong correlation between regular exercise and low CRP levels, which is especially true for men. In one study, investigators found that men who were the most fit tended to have the lowest CRP levels, while those deemed the least fit had the highest levels. The relationship between CRP levels and exercise remained even after adjusting for age and obesity. The risk of elevated CRP decreased incrementally with increasing fitness, with the most fit subjects being 83 percent less likely to have elevated CRP levels than the least fit subjects. The relationship between CRP levels and physical activity in women is probably similar to that in men but is more complicated due to the hormonal changes that occur during menopause.

I am Blood Type B. All of my life I've struggled with chronic constipation and headaches. Now I am noticing that the joints on my fingers are starting to swell. Will the Type B Diet help?

The Blood Type B Diet will certainly do its part. However, you also want to enhance the detoxification pathways in your body by insuring proper eliminative function. The castor oil packs previously described, saunas and dry brushing, and supplements like MSM all help the body process toxins more efficiently, which decreases inflammation.

I am Blood Type B. I work in a hospital as a physical therapist and am constantly exposed to sick patients. A free flu shot is offered annually to employees. Is it beneficial for me to be immunized or take my chances and risk becoming infected with the flu virus?

You are probably better off with the flu (except, of course, a really lethal variant). The protection derived from an actual case is more long-lasting, and Blood Type B can have weird vaccine reactions. Besides, healthy young adults exposed to the flu have symptoms for a few days, but then develop very strong long-term resistance, while the vaccine just protects from a specific strain for a few weeks. Elderberry inhibits neuramidiase, the enzyme used by the influenza virus to attach to the nose and throat, so perhaps a cup of elderberry tea before work would be a good idea.

Blood Type AB

What is glutamine? How essential is it? What are good sources for Blood Type AB?

Glutamine is a protein-building block that serves as a source of fuel for cells lining the intestines. Without it, these cells waste away. It's also used by white blood cells and is important for immune function. In animal research, glutamine has anti-inflammatory effects. Glutamine, in combination with N-acetyl cysteine, promotes the synthesis of glutathione, a naturally occurring antioxidant that is believed to be protective. In the brain, glutamine is converted to glutamic acid, the only alternate source of glucose available to the brain. It provides a ready source of brain fuel for hypoglycemics and helps stave off sugar cravings and hypoglycemic symptoms that develop when blood sugar levels drop too low. Glutamine is also an important source of energy for the nervous system. If the brain is not receiving enough glucose, it compensates by increasing glutamine metabolism for energy—hence, the popular perception of glutamine as "brain food" and its use as a pick-me-up. Glutamine users often report more energy, less fatigue, and better mood.

Glutamine is plentiful in both animal and plant proteins, such as fish, meat, beans, and dairy; and more is synthesized according to need. Be aware, though, that disease, surgery, burn injury, or other acute trauma leads to glutamine depletion with consequent immune dysfunction, intestinal problems, and muscle wasting.

I am Blood Type AB, and I am beginning to suffer from gout. What can be done to lower the chances of a flare-up?

Gout is a form of arthritis that occurs when crystals of uric acid accumulate in a joint, leading to the sudden development of pain and inflammation. Being overweight or having high blood pressure can exacerbate your condition. Be careful not to lose weight too rapidly, however. Because gout is triggered by elevated uric acid levels, and since restriction of calories is known to increase uric acid levels temporarily, it makes sense not to lose weight rapidly.

There is a very clear relationship between diet and gout. Foods that are high in a compound called purine raise uric acid levels in the body. Restricting purine intake can help control uric acid levels and in turn the risk of an attack in individuals susceptible to gout. Foods high in purine are generally protein-rich foods, such as sweetbreads, anchovies, chicken, dried beans and peas, liver and other organ meats, herring, scallops, red meat, and turkey. Avoiding alcohol, particularly beer, or limiting alcohol intake to one drink per day or less can reduce the number of attacks of gout. Refined sugars, including sucrose and fructose, should also be restricted, because they raise uric acid levels.

I am Blood Type AB, and many of the grains are supposed to be all right for my diet. However, after living overseas for some years I apparently developed an allergy to wheat gluten. Because of some digestive problems I was told to cut out of my diet, not just wheat but rye, barley, spelt, and oats as well. Must I really go that drastic route, in your opinion?

Many times, intolerance to a food lectin will develop after a bout of intestinal flu or some other form of gastroenteritis. This has been speculated to be the result of the intestinal inflammation "stripping away" the lining of the intestinal tract, uncovering the base tissue. Normally the gut lining is protected by mucus, the quality of which is determined in large part by your ABO blood type.

This phenomenon supports the old naturopathic wisdom of fasting during acute cases of gastrointestinal disease. Try taking an amino sugar called N-acetyl glucosamine (NAG). This is not glucosamine sulphate, but many health-food stores and catalogs carry it. NAG binds to the agglutinin in wheat so that it cannot react with your digestive lining.

Resources
and Products

General

**National Institute of Arthritis and Musculoskeletal
and Skin Diseases (NIAMS)**
National Institutes of Health
1 AMS Circle
Bethesda, MD 20892–3675
301-495-4484 or 877-22-NIAMS (226-4267)
www.niams.nih.gov

NIAMS provides information about various forms of arthritis and rheumatic diseases and bone, muscle, joint, and skin diseases. It distributes patient and professional education materials and refers people to other sources of information.

Arthritis Foundation
1330 West Peachtree Street
Atlanta, GA 30309
404-872-7100 or 800-283-7800
www.arthritis.org

This is the main voluntary organization devoted to arthritis. The foundation publishes free pamphlets and a monthly magazine for members that provides up-to-date information on arthritis. The foundation can provide physician and clinic referrals. The American Juvenile Arthritis Organization (AJAO) is under the umbrella of the Arthritis Foundation.

Nutrition Research

The Institute for Human Individuality
Southwest College of Naturopathic Medicine
2140 E. Broadway Road
Tempe, AZ 85282
480-858-9100
www.ifhi-online.org

The Institute for Human Individuality is under the 501c3 status of Southwest College of Naturopathic Medicine. Its primary goal is to foster research in the expanding area of human nutrigenomics. Nutrigenomics seeks to provide a molecular understanding for how common dietary chemicals affect health by altering the expression or structure of an individual's genetic makeup. (IFHI is currently conducting a twelve-week randomized, double-blind, controlled trial implementing the Blood Type Diet, to determine its effects on the outcomes of patients with rheumatoid arthritis.)

Products

To purchase supplements mentioned in this book or suggested by your naturopathic physician, your local health-food store is always an excellent resource.

Blood Type–Specific Resources

Dr. Peter D'Adamo

The D'Adamo Naturopathic Center in Stamford, Connecticut blends time-honored natural-healing techniques with state-of-the-art diagnostics. The clinic staff is comprised of naturopathic physicians (NDs) working with medical doctors (MDs), nurses (RNs), and other licensed health professionals, all under the precepts and guidance of Dr. Peter D'Adamo. To find out more or to schedule an appointment, please contact:

The D'Adamo Naturopathic Center
2009 Summer Street
Stamford, CT 06905
203-348-4800

www.dadamo.com

The World Wide Web has proven to be a valuable venue for exploring and applying the tenets of the Blood Type Diet and lifestyle. Since January 1997, hundreds of thousands have visited the site to participate in the ABO chat groups, peruse the scientific archives, share experiences and recipes, and learn more about the science of blood type.

Blood Type Specialty Products and Supplements

North American Pharmacal, Inc., is the official distributor of Blood Type Specialty Products. The product line includes supplements, books, tapes, teas, meal replacement bars, cosmetics, and support material that make eating and living right for your type easier.

North American Pharmacal, Inc.
12 High Street
Norwalk, CT 06851

203-866-7664
Toll free: 1 877-ABO-TYPE (1-877-226-8973)
Fax: 203-838-4066
www.4yourtype.com

Home Blood-Typing Kits

North American Pharmacal, Inc., is the official distributor of Home Blood Type Testing Kits. Each kit costs $9.95 (plus shipping and handling) and is a single-use, disposable, educational device capable of determining one individual's ABO and Rhesus (Rh) blood type. Results are obtained within about four to five minutes. If you have several friends or family members who need to learn their blood types, you will need to order a separate home blood-typing kit for each individual.

The Blood Type Library

The following books are available in bookstores, health-food stores, selected grocery and specialty stores, on the Web, and through North American Pharmacal.

Eat Right 4 Your Type
The Individualized Diet Solution to Staying Healthy, Living Longer, and Achieving Your Ideal Weight
Dr. Peter J. D'Adamo, with Catherine Whitney
G. P. Putnam's Sons, 1996

The original Blood Type Diet ® book, with over 2 million copies sold in more than sixty-five languages.

Cook Right 4 Your Type
The Practical Kitchen Companion to Eat Right 4 Your Type
Dr. Peter J. D'Adamo, with Catherine Whitney
G. P. Putnam's Sons, 1998 (Berkley Trade Paperback, 1999)

Includes over 200 original recipes, thirty-day meal plans, and guidelines for each blood type.

Live Right 4 Your Type
The Individualized Prescription for Maximizing Health, Metabolism, and Vitality in Every Stage of Your Life
Dr. Peter J. D'Adamo, with Catherine Whitney
G. P. Putnam's Sons, 2001

A total health and lifestyle plan based on the individual variations observed for each blood type. Includes new research on the mind-body connection and the importance of blood type secretor status.

Eat Right 4 Your Type Complete Blood Type Encyclopedia
Dr. Peter J. D'Adamo, with Catherine Whitney
Riverhead Books, 2002

The A–Z reference guide for the blood type connection to symptoms, disease, conditions, medications, vitamins, supplements, herbs, and food.

4 Your Type Pocket Guides
Blood Type, Food, Beverage and Supplement Lists
Peter J. D'Adamo, with Catherine Whitney
Berkley Books, 2002

The Eat Right 4 Your Type Portable and Personal Blood Type Guides are pocket-sized and user-friendly. They serve as a handy reference tool while shopping, cooking, and eating out. Each book contains the food, beverage, and supplement list for each blood type plus handy tips and ideas for incorporating the blood type diet into your daily life.

Eat Right 4 Your Baby
The Individualized Guide to Fertility and Maximum Health During Pregnancy, Nursing, and Your Baby's First Year
Dr. Peter J. D'Adamo, with Catherine Whitney
G. P. Putnam's Sons, 2003

An invaluable guide for couples looking to combine the best of naturopathic and blood type science to maximize the health of mother and baby—with practical blood type–specific guidelines for achieving a healthy state before pregnancy, eating and living right during pregnancy, and how to continue in good health during baby's first year.

Dr. Peter J. D'Adamo's Eat Right 4 Your Type Health Library
Diabetes: Fight It with the Blood Type Diet
Cancer: Fight It with the Blood Type Diet
Cardiovascular Disease: Fight It with the Blood Type Diet

Index